A Destroying
Angel

*The Conquest of Smallpox
in Colonial Boston*

Also by
Ola Elizabeth Winslow

American Broadside Verse
Jonathan Edwards, 1703–1758, A Biography
Meetinghouse Hill, 1630–1783
Master Roger Williams
John Bunyan
Samuel Sewall of Boston
John Eliot, "Apostle to the Indians"

For Younger Readers
Portsmouth, The Life of a Town

A Destroying
Angel

The Conquest
of Smallpox
in
Colonial Boston

BY

OLA ELIZABETH WINSLOW

Illustrated with photographs

Houghton Mifflin Company, Boston

1974

First Printing w

Library of Congress Cataloging in Publication Data

Winslow, Ola Elizabeth.
  A destroying angel.

  Bibliography: p.
  1. Smallpox—Boston. I. Title. [DNLM: 1. Small-
pox—History—Massachusetts. 2. Smallpox—Occurrence—
Massachusetts. WC585 W781d 1974]
RC183.5.M4W46   614.5'21'0974461   73–18175
ISBN 0–395–18453–3

Printed in the United States of America

For Blake Cady, M.D.

Honor the physician with the honor due him, according to your need of him, for the Lord created him.

Sirach 38:1

There is a time when success lies in the hands of physicians.

Sirach 38:13, Apocrypha (c. 180 B.C.)

.

On June 2, 1721, as rapidly spreading smallpox became epidemic in Boston, Cotton Mather wrote in his diary:

Because of the destroying Angel standing over the Town, and the grievous Consternation on the Minds of the People, I move the Ministers who are the Lecturers of the City, to turn the next Lecture into a Day of Prayer, that we may prepare to meet our God.

Foreword

"NEW PLANTATIONS, what do they ask of those who hazard them?"
John Winthrop the Younger was once asked.

"All thinges to doe," he wrote, "as in the beginning of the world."

First and second New England generations had answered that
requirement to a remarkable degree, and in so doing had become
men and women who would have seemed strange to their countrymen left behind on the English shore. Third generation sons and
daughters of these early pioneers now had the sense of possessing
the new land, and they were beginning to belong responsibly to it.
Robert Frost was right, deeply right, when at the inauguration of
President Kennedy in Washington, he threw his head back and
shouted into the wind those memorable lines from his poem, "The
Gift Outright:"

> *The land was ours before we were the land's.*
> *She was our land more than a hundred years*
> *Before we were her people . . .*

By 1700 that deeply rooted, invisible, mysterious process of belonging was unconsciously at work in the minds and affections of
third generation sons and daughters.

In outlook and forward reach these men and women of the late
seventeenth and early eighteenth centuries were almost a new race
as compared with the first immigrants to Virginia or New England.
Born during the last two decades of the seventeenth century, their

inheritance had been modified and enriched by two generations of wilderness living. Perseverance, patience, determination, and hope had been sorely tested. This generation would also be pioneers. To the last day of their earthly lives, they would face gigantic tasks of construction and imagination and endure hardships enough. They would also face entirely new problems, and in their attempt to solve them would develop new ideals and capacities. The conquest of disease would be a first imperative.

For centuries before the first immigrants embarked either for Virginia or New England, smallpox had claimed, year by year, its uncounted thousands. In all centers of population it was an endemic disease with only brief respites between one outbreak and the next. Public health measures against it had hardly been imagined. Smallpox came, most men believed, just as tornadoes, lightning, earthquakes, or floods came — as God's test of man's faith, or punishment for his sins. As to safety from infection, that too was in God's hands. The only certainty to which man could hold was that to survive one attack meant that one would never have another. The nature of infection was a deep mystery. What could man do for safety? Nothing, but fast and pray.

It seems fitting in 1973, when the World Health Organization has announced that worldwide smallpox will be eradicated completely from the world before the year's end, to tell the story of the long struggle against this killer and defacer of man, of the devastating epidemics in early Boston, and the consequent discovery of inoculation. In eighteenth-century history inoculation for smallpox marked a new beginning. Science entered the picture, stimulating keener observation, a sharper respect for objective fact, and never-ending experimentation. It reshaped American culture from a new center, leading life and thought out in new directions. In our own deeply troubled, revolutionary, and almost incredibly hopeful twentieth century, this once familiar but now only dimly remembered story takes on a timeless relevance.

Contents

Illustrations

Note

Unfortunately there is no known portrait of Zabdiel Boylston.

A Destroying
Angel
The Conquest of Smallpox in Colonial Boston

An Unprofessional
Medical Background

IN THE EARLY YEARS of the eighteenth century medicine was hardly a profession in America. Indeed, it was little more than a craft or an art to be learned not in a school, but through seven years of apprenticeship in the home of a medical practitioner, who had probably begun to learn what he knew through apprenticeship in his own youth. During this seven-year period (and sometimes less) a boy of thirteen or fourteen was bound to serve his master, keep his secrets, refrain in his conduct from throwing dice, playing cards, attending the theater, frequenting the tavern, or indulging in other traditional vices. He might not leave his master's house without permission, and he might not marry. In return for obedience to all these restraints and for steady industry in all that was required of him from dawn to candlelight, he was promised bed, board, and clothing as well as instruction and training. This system was already centuries old in England, and America brought it over entire.

An apprentice's duties were manifold. He took care of his master's equipment: his mortars, pestles, apothecaries' weights and measures, and all instruments; he cleaned bottles, phials, sponges, sieves, syringes, forceps, cutting and cupping vessels; he powdered dried herbs, ground roots and bark, rolled pills, spread plasters, boiled syrups, made lotions, ointments, salves. Most apprentices also performed various routine chores around the master's house and stable.

On some days an apprentice accompanied his master on his visits to patients, observing and later assisting in the techniques of bleeding, lancing, and bandaging. In time he would be allowed to try his own hand in the treatment of minor injuries under the eye of the master. This close observation and participation was probably the best preparation an immature apprentice received during the seven years of training. Sometimes he stayed on for a time and gained his first independent experience under the guidance of his master, but this was not a requirement. His seven years completed, the apprentice was given an examination, and if he passed it successfully, he was licensed as a practitioner.

His training had been literal, technical, and practical — a training of hand and eye chiefly. What he had missed, he might never know. Colonial practitioners had few books, and he would have been unaware of the perspective books might have begun to supply. The record of medicine through the centuries had been almost a blank page on which was recorded little more than a few names of the great men who had made medicine a profession instead of a craft. The experience of suffering, birth, death, would teach the practitioner much, if he had the sensitivity to learn. His own successes and failures would teach him far more, but a license gained, this was all ahead, years ahead. John Wesley was deeply right when he discovered for himself that "experience and physic grew up together." In colonial America this aphorism became truth.

Even on the literal level, the apprentice system, as preparation for a medical career, had many weaknesses. Perhaps the chief flaw was the lack of uniformly high standards for a candidate's eligibility at the outset of his training and of his promise at the end; even more fault remained in the lack of standard qualifications for the master and of his performance during the years of training. England had attempted, through watchers and searchers, to make a periodic inspection of this technical training, but there was no such effort in New England. Uniform standards at almost any point were totally lacking. They would continue to be so until there were medical schools, hospitals, scientific societies, journals, and an authoritative licensing system to carry out regulations. Some means of continuing a young man's training after he began to practice was imperative. Meanwhile a credulous public was at the mercy of unequally prepared young practitioners, or worse still, of quacks who lived on the fringe of every settlement or traveled from town to town.

Repeatedly laws were passed with intent to rid settlements of such pretenders and to protect the people from injury resulting from low standards of medical education. On May 2, 1649, the Massachusetts legislature passed an act warning midwives, chirurgeons, and physicians that

> Forasmuch as the Law of God allows no man to impaire the Life or Limbs of any Person, but in a judicial way, it is therefore ordered, That no person or persons whatsoever, employed at any time about the bodyes of men, women or children for preservation of life or health as Chirurgeons, Midwives, Physicians or others, presume to exercise or set forth any act contrary to the known approved Rules of Art, in the Mystery and occupation, nor exercise any force, violence or cruelty upon, or towards the body of any, whether young or old (no not in the most difficult or desperate cases) without the advice and consent of patients if they be *compotes,* much less contrary to such advice with the services of such as are skillfull in the same Art.

Severe punishment awaited those who dare attempt whatever was

> to the prejudice or hazard to the life or limbs of man, woman, or child[1]

This law stood on the books, but the situation remained virtually unchanged. Eleven years later another law was passed to regulate the practice of physic and surgery, but it proved to be equally ineffective. Such acts attest the awareness of manifold dangers, but without an authoritative standard behind them, safety for the public had to wait.

Several more lifetimes would pass before notions of health and disease, inherited by their English forebears from medieval times, began to be replaced by more realistic ideas. There was still something more than a tinge of mystery and magic associated with medicine in New England, especially with the curing process. Even John Winthrop the Younger, practical and useful physician that his Connecticut Colony knew him to be, treasured what he thought was a piece of a unicorn's horn in his medicine cabinet. He used it and gained credit thereby. A powder made from the unicorn's horn was said to be miraculous wherever it was applied. Such was the tradition.

His father, John Winthrop, first Governor of Massachusetts Bay Colony, had been promised, upon sailing from Southampton in 1630, an antimonial cup as a parting gift from Matthew Craddock, Governor of the New England Company sponsoring the migration. There is, unfortunately, no evidence that Winthrop received this hopeful token. The fabled cup, made of tin and antimony, had a long tradition behind it and was still believed by many English physicians of that day to possess powers little short of magical.

The theory back of this faith was that after a stated number of hours the wine with which the cup was filled would be impregnated with the healing power that antimony possessed to cure whatever unhealthful symptoms the body was suffering. One Dr. Evans, announcing himself as "Minister and Preacher of God's Word," published a volume in 1634 entitled *The Universall Medicine or the Vertues of the Antimonial Cup.* Evans was also a maker and seller of such cups, and he may have thought to advertise his wares in this array of cures — nineteen in number. They stand as an example of the unspecific nature of disease itself, as then assumed. This view is typically medieval.

The Antimonial Cup or Universal Medicine

1. It keepeth the body from repletion and fulness of humours.
2. It helpeth against all evil effects of the stomach.
3. It cureth all intermittent Agues and burning Fevers.
4. It cureth the green sickness and helpeth against all obstructions.
5. It helpeth the swimming in the head, Madnesse and Frenzie.
6. It preventeth the Stone, the Gout, the Sciatica and other Aches.
7. It is a good Preservative against all Contagions and contagious Diseases.
8. It cureth perfectly Morbus Gallicus and Lues Venerea.
9. It aswageth the Falling Sickness, and all Convulsions.
10. It destroyeth Wormes, and maketh Complexion Faire.
11. It emptieth the Stomache of ill humours; the Liver of Choler; the Spleen of Melancholy; the Pectoral Parts of all hurtfull Humours; the Head and Throat of flegme and rheums, and all distillations.
12. It restoreth appetite lost, and causeth rest to the senses and sleep.
13. It cureth wounds and stancheth Blood.
14. It taketh away Wens and other Excrescences.
15. It purifieth the sight and consumeth the Web and Pearle.
16. It cleaneth and healeth ulcerous sores, and Fistulas.
17. It consumeth rotten and putrified dead flesh.
18. It is excellent against all diseases in Clysters.
19. It aswageth the panic of the Gout.[2]

John Evans also left instructions as to the use of this cup and expressed protest against those who misused it. "And if you finde not yourselfe afterwards more hungrie, lively, and cheerful, beleeve me not." Antimony was one of the first metallic substances used in seventeenth-century practice. John Winthrop, Jr., used it extensively in his Connecticut medical practice.

Three manuscript sheets bearing the date 1634 and labelled *Recipes, for my worthy friend Mr. Winthrop,* found among the Winthrop papers owned by the Massachusetts Historical Society, suggest the substitution of simple and easily accessible materials for the cure of common ills instead of the rare or nonexistent talismans of medieval legend. These recipes are a fair example of medical prescriptions commonly used in New England during the middle years of the seventeenth century, particularly if help from a physician or an apothecary shop was not available.

For the Stone

Make a concoction of maiden hayre, fennel and parsley root. Lette him drink great quantities. But first lett him drink 2 or 3 ounces of ye Oyle of Almonde newly extracted or more. Or let him swallow a quarter of a pound of new butter made into round bullets, and cast into fayre water to harden them.

For the yellow jaundice or Jaunders

Boyle a quart of sweet milk, dissolve therein as much baysalt, or fine salt-petre as shall make it brackish to taste; and putting Saffron in a fine linen clout, rubb it into ye Milke, until ye Milke be very yellow and give it ye patient to drinke.

For Paines in ye Brest or Limmes

Weare a Wild Catte skin on ye pla^{ce} grieved.

For old Sores

St. John's Wort pound it small, mingle it with as much quick lime, Pour on it rainwater to cover 6 fingers deep, stir it well once a day for a month, Filter and reserve the water in a broad earthen vessel for your use. Put it in the sun. Wash the sore with it. It cures wonderfully.

For a broken bone or a joynt dislocated, to knit them

Take ye barke of Elm, or witch-hazel; cut away ye outward part. Cutte ye Inward redd barke small, and boyle it in water, till it be thick that it will rope; pound it very well, and lay it on hott, barke and all upon ye Bone or Joynt, and tye it on with the Musilage hot and bole Armenian (a soft clayey earth of a bright red color). Make a plaster and lay it on.

This list closes with "these receipts are all experimented."[3] There is less of marvel in them than in many other remedies of the mid-century, suggesting perhaps that the physician offering them was on his way to be a realist. Dr. Oliver Wendell Holmes once made an unsuccessful attempt to discover his name.

The unspecific character of most early New England remedies need surprise no one, for until 1800 very few diseases had been identified and recognized by their own individual symptoms. Small-pox and yellow fever, yes; malaria, not always; respiratory and intestinal irritations, which were chiefly responsible for the high death rate, had only this loose classification. Diseases must be discovered before cures could be found, and that time was not yet.

Basic to medical theory was the notion of the four humors: blood, phlegm, bile (yellow and black), being responsible for the health of the "body system" as it was called. If these four humors, or body fluids as they were thought to be, were in proper proportion with each other and were functioning properly, the "body system" was in health; if not, it was diseased, and remedy would come by depletion. Hence bleeding, purging, sweating, would free the body system of the poisons that were making it unhealthy. Almost always, the first and most important of these techniques was bleeding. Age-old and standard, it was applied whatever the apparent difficulty of the patient, child or adult. As to quantity, that was left to the physician entirely.

Some of the more fantastic of the widely known English remedies were lost on the way to America or survived only as conversation pieces, but once in a while one appears unexpectedly. Sir Kenelm Digby's "sympathetic powder" came by legend only, as he kept the ingredients a secret and insisted on administering the magic himself in the homeland.

This magic formula had been given to Sir Kenelm — he said — by a Carmelite priest who had learned it either in India or Persia. For twenty years thereafter it was known and heralded in England as Sir Kenelm's. He used it in the healing of open wounds — sword wounds in particular. A discourse on this powder, translated from the French into English, reports the case of James Howell, a friend of Sir Kenelm's, and one of the favorites of James I. Wounded in his attempt to separate two friends in a duel, James Howell had received a severe cut on his hand. The king's physician was called, but his service brought no relief. Howell's hand swelled, and he was in great pain.

Sir Kenelm was then summoned. He asked for two pails of water, put a handful of powder in one of them, and washed the injured hand in the clear water of the other pail, using the garter of James Howell in dressing the wound. This process completed, he dropped the garter into the pail containing the powder. Instantly James Howell's pain ceased. When Sir Kenelm took the bloodstained garter out of the pail, the pain returned again. The sword that had caused the wound was then greased and the sympathetic powder was sprinkled on it. There was no contact between the patient and the garter or the water into which it had been placed. During the day-time a basin containing the garter was kept in a closet; at night it was placed in the chimney corner. The temperature was kept moderate else the wounded man suffered pain. The powder, a sulphate of various minerals, had been dissolved in water and recrystallized in the sun, the secret supposedly being that the sun's rays extracted the spirits of the blood and the powder that were attracted. When this secret was revealed, the powder lost its potency, and Sir Kenelm had the wisdom to keep silent thereafter.[4] A modern skeptic might dare to suggest that cleansing the wound in clear water and then leaving it alone might possibly have given nature a chance in the healing. But magic in medicine would have lost a good story.

Sir Kenelm is also credited with sending John Winthrop the Younger a recipe for using crab's eyes as a healing ingredient, but whether or not he used them successfully seems not to have been recorded.

There were various recipes that gave frogs a similar honor to crabs. Dr. John Wadsworth of Duxbury had several magic potions made from both frogs and toads — especially for the curing of cancer — since they were believed to possess the power to draw poison out of affected parts. One of these recipes reads thus:

> Take three frogs. Put them in a deep earthen basin, cover them with sweet oil, and put the basin in a hot oven for a quarter of an hour. Draw off the remaining oil. Dip a tourniquet in it and apply this to the cancer.

Wadsworth also had two other recipes for cancer cure as follows:

> Apply a toad cut in half two or three times a week. This will draw out the sharp, hot, cancerous poison. You can cure any cancer with it.
>
> Cool the patient's blood with a portion of Epsom salt. The patient's constant drink must be cancer-root tea and Dinelybit tea.[5]

Such marvels were numerous and the memory of them tenacious enough so that the physician must somehow rid the patient of the hopes they had raised before he opened his satchel and began a more scientific treatment.

Until well through the first century, most medicines in America were chiefly botanical — herbs being particularly popular. New England's sumac, elderberry, saffron, snake root were considered good "for bringing out the measles and chicken-pox," as well as curing snakebite. Sassafras and witch hazel healed bruises and sprains. Most of these were grown in the garden and used widely. For generations the English had been accustomed to searching woods and fields for medical plants, and they were experienced in finding and preparing them. The old adage, "Find the herb where the disease occurs," had been put to frequent use in New England as well as in the homeland. Indian knowledge and experience had added new specifics to be sought. Households fortunate enough to possess an herbal found abundant need to consult it, as did their borrowing neighbors, with the result that this precious book was often not in its place on the kitchen shelf.

Quantities of the medicine suitable for a dose were all by rule of thumb. One finds such phrases as "a large quantity," the "bigth of a walnut," enough from which "to lie on the point of a penknife." A "pretty bunch of flowers" would be sufficient to make a lotion.

The first wonder drug of the century, discovered not by research but by accident, was cinchona bark, also called "Peruvian bark," but more commonly only "the bark." Native to the region of the Andes and cultivated in India and Java, it yielded quinine and other alkaloids. Actually effective for certain fevers, it was customarily given for all, as though what helped one would help the others. Debate often waxed lively over which bark, the red or the brown, would be more effective, but custom was usually to try both. First-generation settlers had come well furnished with enduring memories of folk medicine. Next came home remedies, blessed also in large supply. Magic, astrology, occult practices, and prayer completed the available resources. It would be a long time before men gave up their hospitable response to fantastic cures.

During the earlier decades of the great migration to New England, European scientists were beginning to give men a new view of themselves and the world in which they lived. Old wives' tales had taken care of the earth's mysteries for a long time, but resources of ancestral folklore could not deal successfully with man's unanswered questions in the new day that was almost at hand.

Some of the men in the van of the illustrious company of scientists had already announced their new findings; some had finished their work and had gone. William Harvey had published his discovery of the circulation of the blood before the *Mayflower* arrived in Plymouth harbor. Francis Bacon, "Trumpeter of his time," was asleep before Plymouth was six years old. Kepler died in 1630, the year of Boston's founding. During these same early years of the new century, Galileo had faced the Inquisition for declaring publicly his agreement with Copernicus that, contrary to Psalm 93, the sun, not the earth, was the center of the universe and that the earth revolved around it. Blind and imprisoned after his trial, Galileo lived on until 1642, which was the birth year of Sir Isaac Newton, who more than any other man would awaken the grandsons of New England's first generation to their lifelong pursuit of science.

A large new area of discovery was just ahead, and the young men of the third American generation would move into it. The pace would be slow and every step would be challenged by the ancient tradition. Microscopes would begin to uncover long-hidden secrets and to excite hopes of what stronger lenses would presently reveal. The rudiments of chemical analysis would begin to show that the four humors were not simple fluids but that each was a complex system within itself. Better trained medical men would come to New England and their influence would be felt. Third generation young men looking toward a medical career were ready to respond to the new world of experimentation that had been largely unknown to the pastor-physicians whom they would replace.

II

A Half Century
of Pastor-Physicians

THE DUAL ROLE of preaching and healing arose naturally among English university students in the early years of the century. Particularly during the supremacy of William Laud, Bishop of London in 1628, and Archbishop of Canterbury after 1638, nonconforming young men who were looking toward the ministry as a profession knew they would have no chance of securing a living in the established church, but that medical practice would still be open to them. Accordingly, they added anatomy and physiology to their study of theology, and on taking their degree, were eligible to practice medicine if they so desired.

One of these young men, John Fiske of Emanuel College, wrote to John Winthrop that "seeing the danger of the Times," when the silencers were hard upon him, he "had changed his profession of divinitie into physic, was licensed therein." But divinity was still his first choice, and when he saw a chance to preach in America, he took ship in disguise and escaped to New England. For a time he kept a school in his own home and practiced medicine while helping Hugh Peter in his pulpit. Later Fiske preached briefly in Wenham, and then moved to Chelmsford, where for twenty years he continued to dispense medicines for the body along with his care of the soul.[1] His story can be matched many times in the 1630s by those of other young university graduates who arrived in the first ships. Some of them practiced the two professions in the opposite order and had to wait ten or twenty years before the pulpit could be all their care.

Most of them had to be content with being a preacher on Sunday and a physician on weekdays.

More often than not, if an appointment to preach in a newly settled village came quickly, the young clergyman found himself the only university man in the settlement, and the only resident with any acquaintance whatever with medicine. Inevitably illness came, and his skill and knowledge, meager though they were, were all that anyone had to offer. His people needed him, and their importunity gave him no choice.

His English training as a university student gave such a man no direct contact with illness but was entirely theoretical. He had "read" medicine, as the saying went, and through this reading had gained some knowledge of anatomy and physiology, some acquaintance with drugs, but no knowledge whatever about their preparation and use. The newly qualified clergyman-doctor had never rolled a pill or spread a plaster. He had no experience in a hospital, had never made a diagnosis or treated a patient. When suddenly faced with the reality of suffering, possibly with death too near not to be recognized as imminent, he put his theoretical knowledge to work and learned fast.

In his university "reading" of medicine, he had most likely begun with the classics — probably first with Hippocrates (c. 460–c. 370 B.C.). In his youth, says Plato, Hippocrates came to Protagoros, "that mighty wise man, to learn the science and knowledge of human life." About what Hippocrates learned and practiced during his life we know very little, but his name endures in the professional "credo" which even today is still prescribed by many boards of medical advisors as the formula of admission to medical practice.

Seventeenth-century students would have carried away from their reading of Hippocrates a few fundamental ideas — perhaps the strongly and repeatedly emphasized concept that disease proceeds from natural causes, not from witches and demons, and the belief in the healing power of nature. Above all, they would have ab-

sorbed Hippocrates's persistent insistence upon careful, direct examination and observation as the essentials for medical knowledge.
Hippocrates had come to these fundamental concepts through a lifetime of precise and careful observation which he relentlessly demanded of his students.

English medical students would also have been led directly to
Galen (A.D. 130–200), who called himself a disciple of Hippocrates's, and who like Hippocrates was a philosopher as well as an
observer and experimenter. All English medical students read Galen
in their own tongue, and if they owned a medical text, it would have
been Galen's work from one of the several editions available. Above
all others, Galen was the authority to be consulted — an authority
that was definitive until the early eighteenth century, when at last it
began to be questioned.

Precisely what seventeenth-century medical students would have
been advised to read from Galen is not known specifically, but one
hopes they did not miss his discussions and diagrams of the heart. If
these portions were studied, students could hardly have missed the
stimulus Galen provided toward direct observation, attested to by
Harvey's 1613 preliminary announcement of the circulation of the
blood. Harvey (1658–1757) was an elder contemporary of these
students and though his proclamation was met by bleak disbelief by
the older medical men, it was a news item no seventeenth-century
medical student could ignore, not only as a possible fact, but probably also as an example of what direct observation had brought to
pass.

How indeed could Galen have missed discovering the circulation
of the blood himself centuries before, one might dare to ask. He had
recognized the two systems, that of the veins and of the arteries. He
had described their differences and perceived that they could communicate. He had also recognized the ebb and flow of the blood and
the vibrating force in the walls and valves of the heart. What he
did not see was that the heart itself is a pump as well as the source

of animal heat. His medical students of the 1620s and 1630s might have recognized that his principle of direct observation had brought him to the conclusions illustrated in his diagram of the heart. They would live long enough to realize that later steps in direct observation would also explain Harvey's discovery.

With their further reading of medicine beyond the classical period and possibly a brief experience in a dissecting academy, New England pastor-physicians came armed with at least a modicum of theoretical knowledge that village emergencies might make effective in practical application. As his congregation became his patients as well as Sabbath listeners, there is no doubt that he faced a barricade of superstition, ignorance, and adherence to a long tradition of folk custom that would threaten to defeat his best efforts to apply even the slightest scientific methods. But helpless as he might be to change this situation, and ill-prepared as he would discover he was, experience would give him confidence as he struggled to apply the little he knew. A few diaries of these young practitioners could tell us more than we shall ever know of this most important early chapter of American medical history.

These pastor-physicians soon became a numerous company. At first entirely English-trained, their ranks soon included a few New England sons as well, for Harvard College began to offer lectures on anatomy and physiology according to the English university plan. During the early years a few English boys came over, some of them remaining a few years as pastor-physicians before going home. For the most part, the members of the group are unknown personalities, except for a chance reference to their skill or to some special talent they may have exhibited. From such items their story expands a little.

For example, Giles Firmin, whose ministry dates from 1637, was also the first formal instructor in medicine in Massachusetts Bay Colony. He had come in 1630 as a young boy in company with his father, Giles Firmin, on Winthrop's flagship, the *Arbella.* After his father's death within the year, Giles Firmin, Jr., returned to England to continue his studies in medicine at the university. His course completed, he came back to New England where he preached and practiced medicine.

Testimony as to his teaching medicine to American students comes from a letter of John Eliot, missionary to the Indians, written to Thomas Shepard, September 24, 1627, in connection with Eliot's plea for a better education for "young students in physic who have only theoretical knowledge and are forced to fall to practice before they ever see an Anatomy made or are duely trained in making Experiments." Then came the name of Giles Firmin, "for we never had but one Anatomy in the country, which Mr. Giles Firmin made and read upon very well."[2] One month later, the General Court record reads:

> We conceive it very necessary yt such as studies Physic, or Chirurgy may have liberty to read Anatomy and to anatomize once in four years some malefactor, in case there be such as the Courts shall know of.[3]

Anatomy is an obsolete word for *skeleton,* and John Eliot's statement that Giles Firmin himself made the skeleton he read upon suggests that he made it by dissection, for which his instruction may have been acquired at an English dissecting academy during his own university period. Where he lectured on the skeleton he made is not stated, but very probably it was at Harvard.

Thomas Thacher was another pastor-physician who has been remembered for a quite different important reason. As a boy his nonconformist convictions were already so strong that he refused to attend an English university because of the orthodox subscription he knew would be required of him before he could receive his degree. He came to America and studied in the home of Charles Chauncy of Scituate, one of the most learned men of the first generation. At that time Chauncy was minister in Scituate and also a physician. Later he became the second President of Harvard College.

Under his tutelage Thomas Thacher became proficient not only in Greek and Latin, but also in Hebrew, Arabic, and Syriac. For twenty years he preached and practiced medicine in Weymouth, then moved to Boston, where he established a second medical reputation and was later called to be the first pastor of the newly gathered Old South Church where he served until his death in 1678. In 1677 when smallpox was epidemic in Boston, he published a broadside entitled *A Brief Rule to Guide the Common-People of New England how to order themselves and theirs in the Small Pocks, or Measels.*[4] The content was not originally Thomas Thacher's, rather it seemed to be a simple paraphrase of various details in the writings of Thomas Sydenham, an English physician (1624–1689), whose publications include a book, *Dissertation epistolaris* (1682), in which his observations on smallpox are printed. However, if not original, Thacher's broadside was significant in medical history as it was the first publication of its kind in the colonies.

Despite the crowded broadside page which made this memorable guide difficult to follow, it was apparently widely read in the grimness of the 1677 outbreak. It includes common sense suggestions such as Thacher himself had doubtless followed in his treatment of smallpox patients — simple remedies and unceasing care to give nature a chance to affect a cure without medicines. Such was the core of his advice. Abstain from flesh and wine, he said, "and for food, water-gruel, water-potage, boil'd apples, and milk sometimes for a Change, but the coldness taken off." Almost any household could have supplied what he recommended. The simplicity and common sense quality in these instructions suggest a realistic point of view perhaps true for many of this all but unknown company of pastor-physicians whose work was so badly needed when trained doctors did not exist in sufficient number.

One of the best-known names of men in this group is that of

Michael Wigglesworth, but his fame comes neither from his preaching nor from his medical skill. Posterity remembers him as the brimstone poet of *The Day of Doom*,[5] owned in its day by every thirty-fifth person in New England — a record not equalled by any book except the Bible since that time. More amazing still, this poem was memorized through all of its two hundred and twenty-four sulphurous stanzas by many score of these owners. The jingling ballad meter and lurid doggerel tone not only invited to singsong memorization, but also probably awakened the learners of the torments of hell in time for them to escape the doom.

Michael Wigglesworth himself, "a feeble shadow of a man," was a lifetime sufferer from many ills, but so tender of heart that in spite of Calvin he consigned "reprobate Infants" who had died too soon to be given the grace of baptism, to be carried "from the womb to the tomb" and placed in "the easiest room in Hell." "A Little Piece, Written by a Fool," Wigglesworth called his best seller, and probably meant what he said when he wrote, "Reader, I am a Fool." Modern readers, if they stay with this poem through as many as a dozen pages, will probably admit the vigor of these blazing stanzas as the last trumpet sounds, and, "Horror the world doth fill."

> *The mountains smoke, the hills are shook,*
> *The earth is rent and torn,*
> *As if she should be clear dissolved,*
> *Or from the center borne.*
> *The sea doth roar, forsakes the shore*
> *and shrinks away for fear,*
> *The wild beasts flee into the sea*
> *as soon as he draws near.*

Calvinism deserved this poem, and it could not have been written except by one to whom the inescapable doom was literal truth.

Wigglesworth seems also to have been something of a student in medicine to judge from the testimony of his bookshelves, which, from a total of eighty titles, held eighteen volumes dealing with medical subjects and these eighteen indicate a considerable body of specialized knowledge. Physic was a lifelong interest with him, and fairly early in his career, he had worried lest this persistent interest "might withdraw" his attention from theology. Apparently he escaped this danger or outlived it, as a brother minister, John Rogers, preacher in Ipswich, failed to do when his "disposition for medieval studies caused him to abate of his Labours in the pulpit." Perhaps the fact that soon afterward Rogers was elected President of Harvard College may have saved him from guilt in withdrawing from theology, but as to that we shall never know, for he died within the year of his election.

Another pastor-physician, Edward Taylor, of remote Westfield, Massachusetts, had to wait until the twentieth century before it was discovered that in his lifetime labors of preaching and healing in his small congregation, he had found time to write an unsuspected volume of metaphysical poetry without parallel in America's literary story. Taylor was a man of scholarly tastes and untiring zeal in their pursuit who had an imaginative life totally unknown and unguessed by those with whom he labored. For fifty-eight years this man of endearing personal qualities ministered to his congregation as preacher and healer. Once a year he made a horseback journey to the Harvard commencement, met his friends, bought a book or two, and returned to this pioneer company, to which he had belonged since he was a young college graduate.

The distinction of his poetry lies in its kinship with those we call the English metaphysical poets, Herbert and Crashaw. Though he joined these men a century late and differed from them in material and method, Taylor's elevation and art were a match for those of Herbert and Crashaw. Like them, he reached for the unattainable in religious ecstasy and expressed his experience in elaborate conceits and far-fetched metaphors. His knowledge of botany was extensive and his use of it medically, according to Nicholas Culpepper's *Directory,* gave him the basic analogies for his religious poetry. Health for the soul was achieved by a purging with "Palma Christi for my sin," healing with "Plastrum Gratiae Dei" and "Unguent Apostolorum." In almost all Taylor's poems one finds the plants of his woods and fields, and always the analogy of God's dispensatory to "sweeten" the art of physical healing with the miracle of divine ministration.

A few lines from "Meditation 62" may illustrate. He finds the text for this meditation in the Song of Solomon, or Canticles as he called it, 1:12, "while the king sitteth at his table, my spikenard sendeth forth the smell therof." Bid to this solemn feast, the poet sings,

> I'le surely come; Lord, fit mee for this feast:
>   Purge me with Palma Christi for my sin.
> With Plastrum Gratiae Dei, or at least
>   Unguent Apostolorum healing bring.
>   Give me thy Sage and Savory: me dub
> With Golden Rod, and with Saint Johns Wort good.
>
> Root up my Henbain, Fawnbain, Divells bit,
>   My Dragons, Chokewort, Crosswort, Ragwort, vice:
> And set my knot with Honeysuckles, stick
>   Rich Herb-a-Grace, and Grains of Paradise,
>   Angelica, yea Sharons Rose the best,
>   And Herba Trinitatis in my breast.
>
>   . . .
>
> Whether I at thy Table Guest do sit,
>   And feed my tast, or Wait, and Fat mine Eye
> And Eare with Sights and Sounds, Heart Rapture fit:
>   My Spicknard breaths its sweet perfumes with Joy.
>   My heart thy Vial with this spicknard fill
>   Perfumed praise to thee then breath it will.

If the readers cannot understand this highly wrought imagery now and then, no one would fail to know what he meant when he sent "Wagonloads of love" to God, called sinners "Jayle Birds," or saw Satan "with goggling Eyes." Perhaps Edward Taylor is not to be explained, but he can be read with delight and his divine dispensatory need be no enigma at all. As a poet, his touch is alchemical.[6]

Gersholm Bulkeley (1635–1713), son of Peter Bulkeley, first generation preacher of Concord, Massachusetts, exhibited the vehemence of his forebears in a new direction. He was not motivated by zeal for orthodoxy that had made his father the ruthless persecutor of Anne Hutchinson at her trial for heresy in 1637, but by a ferocious loyalty to English monarchy — "the best form or kind of government" — and an eloquent contempt for the substitute rule of his countrymen after the overthrow of Governor Andros. Gersholm Bulkeley had been living the life of pastor-physician and unusually skillful surgeon in Colchester, Connecticut, until the outbreak of King Philip's War found a new role for him, that of chaplain and surgeon in the Continental army. His bravery and the success of his surgery brought him a citation in the form of a vote of thanks from the General Court of Connecticut Colony. He was also made a member of the Council of War and at one time commanded a small company of soldiers in an attack. Wounded, he returned to his parish, moved to Wethersfield, and later left the ministry but continued to practice medicine and surgery until after the expulsion of Andros, when he became Justice of the Peace for Hartford County, Connecticut. His pamphlet, *Objections,* later reprinted under the title, *Will and Doom,*[7] is the first American expression of anti-democratic conviction in print. It seems a lawyer's utterance, as indeed it was, for Bulkeley was deeply grounded in law as well as in theology. He built a strong case for monarchy and scorched his opponents in their rebellion against the king, which, as he saw it, was rebellion against God and "like the sin of witchcraft." "The king's government was better with us than ever it was under your government,"

he asserted again and again, with blistering epithets to his countrymen "for their Tumults, Insurrections, Rebellions, Riots, Sedition,
and Treason" during the stormy period of Andros.

From one parish to the next, these pastor-physicians left behind
them a record not only of six-day readiness to keep their congregations in physical health, but also of considerably narrowing the
natural gap between pulpit and pew doubtless by their friendly
ministrations. To have eased pain, cured a sick child, saved a life,
added another dimension to the minister's role in colonial life and
village thought. These men did not advance the cause of medicine.
They held the fort during a time when they were needed, and here
and there among them one finds a man of memorable stature beyond preaching and healing.

In various ways the most illustrious man in the long line of pastor-
physicians was Jared Eliot, son of Joseph Eliot, and grandson of
John Eliot of Massachusetts. Taught medicine by his father after
his graduation from Yale in 1706, Jared Eliot was the lifetime pastor at Killingworth, Connecticut, a parish from which, during forty
years of service, he was seldom, if ever, absent on preaching days.
On all other days he was riding on horseback throughout Connecticut Colony, achieving the reputation of being the best physician the
settlers knew, and also being so busy with his other projects, which
had nothing to do with either preaching or healing, that it is no
wonder to read as a footnote to his life that he slept less than any
other man in Connecticut. He was a man of deep and wide learning
and a linguist; he was particularly abreast of scientific achievements
in many directions and the practical application of these discoveries.

In addition to preaching and healing, Eliot wrote a series of agri-
cultural essays growing out of his own experimentation with the
draining of swamps, deep plowing, and rotation of crops. His attempt to transfer scientific theory to agriculture was the first of its
kind in the new world and opened the eyes of his fellow farmers to
new possibilities not only in America, but also in England, where his

essays proved widely influential. He introduced the cultivation of the white mulberry to Connecticut, made a beginning with the culture of silkworms and the manufacture of silk. In this venture he had in mind an industry that New Englanders might follow during the long winter season between sowing and reaping of crops in the field. He also owned and operated an iron foundry and shortly before his death he was concerned with the possibility of making steel out of a certain black sand he found along the Connecticut shore. The range of his ideas, his high standard of performance, and the liveliness of his inventive imagination in various fields made him unique for his day.[8] When he died in 1663, a new era had already begun. He was the last of the pastor-physicians who wrote a significant chapter in New England's story of medicine stretching back for a half century.

In a still wider sense Eliot is seen as one in the distinguished group of America's first scientists remembered not only for his concrete achievements, but also for something of future promise that these suggested. In the phrase of his contemporary, J. Hector St. John Crèvecoeur, author of *Letters from an American Farmer,* he might well be that "new man" of European descent, but different from a European, one of "a new race of men, whose labours and posterity will some day cause great changes in the world." Jared Eliot's life story from beginning to end gives us many clues as to how Americans have developed from a race of farmers into the originators of our complex way of life, indeed, our total culture and character as a nation.

III

Five Major Outbreaks in One Lifetime Span

TERROR OF SMALLPOX and deaths from it had been part of English life for centuries before the first settlements were attempted in New England. For most passengers who climbed aboard John Winthrop's fleet of seventeen ships in 1630 some portion of this long travail was part of their own ancestral record. For others the trial was as brief and recent as the last two years when London and the countryside for miles around had been held in heavy siege. If these men and women thought that life in a hemisphere far to the west would mean freedom from this scourge of the generations, they would soon learn otherwise.

On the Atlantic coast the West Indies would be almost a neighbor, and these islands from which many trading ships would come were known centers of smallpox infection. Neither New England nor any other geography was safe. Smallpox was a fact of life, as inexorable as the changes of the seasons.

Most adults among the earliest passengers on these seventeen ships to arrive in New England had already acquired immunity from smallpox infection in an earlier attack, probably in childhood. Throughout the seventeenth century smallpox was still regarded as a childhood disease and was frequently confused with measles. In a general outbreak the infection of children was almost without exception, and when the outbreak ended, few families could report an unbroken circle, for mortality figures usually ran highest among the young.

Precise figures are hard to come by for the first half of the seventeenth century and earlier, but after the compilations of Dr. James Jurin, Secretary of the Royal Society in London, the magnitude of England's tragic loss began to be apparent. Looking backward over whatever records were available, he estimated that for the preceding forty-five years at least one fourteenth of the total population in and about London had died of smallpox. For a group of towns of nearly equal size in this territory, the ratio had been one death in every five; for the army, one in every four. Later compilations from 1631 to 1665 showed one death from smallpox in every eleven.[1] The toll of unrecorded deaths from all the wars of English history through the centuries to 1630, could they be known, probably would not begin to match this loss.

With a share of these unknown totals part of nearly every family history, and with the heavy losses of the 1628 outbreak just behind them, the first immigrants to the American Boston set sail. No one on any of these seventeen ships could have been surprised when he learned that smallpox had come on board with them. Two of Francis Higginson's children were infected and one child died. The infection spread, but when the voyage was over, Francis Higginson could report, "But thanks be to God, none dyed but my own child." Few other ships could report only one death. A 1631 passenger wrote, "We were wondrous sick as we came at Sea with the Small Poxe." Fourteen deaths were reported for that ship.

During the first four years of the Boston settlement there were a few cases as infected ships came in but no general outbreak until 1634 when Dutch ships brought the disease to Indians along the Connecticut River. According to William Bradford's report, "Multitudes dyed." They had no immunity from previous outbreaks. Sporadic cases continued to be reported year after year in Boston and in most other early settled towns of the neighborhood. Fast days were appointed together with days of humiliation, always with a sermon detailing the local calendar of local sins with penance to match in the hope that God's anger might be appeased before the blow struck. Man was the offender and also the victim. God sent the smallpox.

Records are scant as to the details of these annual visitations, but as one senses from diaries, journals, town and church records, line-a-day pages in the annual extant almanacs, the impression grows that smallpox had been accepted almost perfunctorily as one of the hazards of life along with all the other disasters of the year — tornadoes, floods, locusts, Indian raids, and fires by night. In 1638 spotted fever increased the severity of the outbreak in Dedham; in 1648 whooping cough in Scituate and Barnstable brought death to many children ill with the smallpox; in 1666 John Hull's diary reported that "as the cold increased, so did the smallpox and became very mortal." Again and again in these private records, one reads only that "it was a very dying time."

In 1675 Cotton Mather prophesied in a sermon that "very soon God will lift up his hand against Boston." Apparently he did so in the very serious outbreak of 1677–1678, which cost the town many useful leaders. One grim moment of this visitation came on September 30, 1677, when thirty persons died in one day. Stricter quarantine was applied and travel to nearby towns forbidden. It was during this outbreak that Thomas Thacher, soon to become minister of the Old South Church, published his broadside, *A Brief Rule to Guide the Common-People of New-England how to order themselves and theirs in the Small Pocks, or Measels.* This was the first medical treatise published in America. It was probably widely used during this outbreak and remembered for a long time.

Another serious outbreak came in 1689–1690 with the arrival of a ship from the Barbados. This time the infection extended as far as New York on the south and well into Canada on the north. Three hundred and twenty deaths were reported from New Hampshire. A paragraph in the first and only issue of New England's first newspaper, *Publick Occurrences,* appearing on September 20, 1690, and suppressed at once, reads:

The smallpox which has been raging in Boston, after a manner very extraordinary, is now very much abated. It is thought that far more have been sick of it than were visited with it, when it raged so much twelve years ago. Nevertheless it has not been so mortal. The number of them that have dyed in Boston by this last visitation is perhaps not half as many as fell by the former. The time of its being most mortal was in the months June, July, and August when "sometimes in the Congregation on Lord's Day there would be Bills desiring Prayers for above a hundred sick." It seized upon all sorts of People that came in the way of it, even infected children in the bowels of their mothers that had themselves undergone the Disease many years ago; some were born full of the Distemper. 'Tis not easy to translate the Trouble and Sorrow that poor Boston has felt by this Epidemical Contagion. But we hope that it will be pretty well extinguished by that Time twelve Month since it first began to spread.[2]

There was another serious outbreak in 1702 when scarlet fever came with the smallpox. On July 4 Cotton Mather wrote in his diary, "It began to spread." On October 22, "It is on every side of us," and in late December, "More than fourscore people, were in this black Month of December, carried from this Town to their long Home." Three of his own children survived this attack, or as he put it, "came alive out of the fiery Furnace of the Small Pox which almost consumed them."[3] His wife also died at this time but not of smallpox. After 1702 there was a nineteen-year respite before the most severe outbreak of the century in 1721–1722, the sixth since the founding of Boston.

From the arrival of the Winthrop fleet, 1630 to 1632, to 1702 had been a Biblical lifetime span — three score years and ten. Boston's five major outbreaks had been tragically costly. In addition and in almost every year there had been outbreaks in the small neighboring settlements and in fishing villages along the shore,

minor only in the numbers involved. Hardly twelve months had
passed anywhere in the whole region without causing manifold
terrors and leaving mourning families. By 1721, after nearly a century of alternating fear and brief periods of respite, it would seem
that very little had been done by way of public health protection and
planning against the next inevitable attack. In this area experience
had been a slow teacher.

In fairness, however, one may answer: lacking even the beginnings of knowledge and understanding as to the nature of infection, what could they do? Hundreds of cases had made the symptoms familiar, but how did the disease enter the body in the beginning? Through the air they breathed, the water they drank, the food
they ate, or only by the touch of one infected? Human eyes did not
reveal the secret, and what other means did they possess?

Perhaps they had done all they could do. In addition to establishing days of prayer, humiliation, and fasting, they had observed a
few precautions. As early as 1648, upon hearing of "a large Disease"
in the West Indies, the General Court had ordered that all ships
from that area drop anchor three miles from Boston harbor and allow "no persons or goods from the ship to be brought ashore without the permission of three members of the Council." The mention
of *goods* suggests that already there was suspicion of danger from
clothing, baggage, bales of cotton, or other merchandise on board
There is record of ships being detained while goods on board could
be carried to some "distant point" or "well aired," and always with
the caution "none to entertain persons coming from the ship." This
precaution was defeated in 1649 by the canceling of an order pro-
viding for a permanent house for the storing of such goods "well
outside the harbor" because "it hath pleased God to stay the sickness
there."

There were also selectmen's orders during times of infection for-
bidding the airing of bedding in the front yard or along the turn-
pike. All such articles were to be brought to a stated place where

they were guarded day and night. Some awareness of danger no doubt called for these attempted safeguards which were in themselves scant enough protection, and as was also the later requirement in the stagecoach era that passengers and baggage in coaches between New York and Boston be "smoked" at stated points immediately outside each city. One may imagine that this intended guarantee of safety from infection would at least be remembered until the next stagecoach journey. In 1717 a small hospital, crudely equipped, was provided on Spectacle Island in Boston Harbor, in which incoming passengers on infected ships could be held for examination or cared for during their illness, but this accommodation was quickly too small for any but occasional cases.

Even these few precautions and safeguards appear to have been casually observed except during an outbreak. There is record of one captain of an incoming ship who gave false answer as to illness on board, of another who admitted illness, but did not know what it was. Other ships passed too briefly for proper answer to inquiry to be made and then advanced to the dock without waiting for permission to do so. Defeat of almost any safeguard in advance of an outbreak, particularly after a nineteen-year interval — as was true for the 1721 outbreak — was due to the fact that in such a period a whole generation of children had grown up without any chance of immunity resulting from an earlier attack. Also very few of the adult population had any active memory of the reality of terror in a town-wide infection or of the procedures necessary in such a crisis. Awareness of danger was meager in all directions in 1721. Then inevitably crisis came.

Through each of the preceding five outbreaks, Boston had the protection of a few medical men. Too few by far, but from the earliest years, settlers had come with some assurance of medical care. Lambert Wilson, a chirurgeon, had come with John Endicott to Salem in 1628. He was under contract with the English company responsible for the migration, and had agreed to serve the Company and the other Planters that live in the Plantation for three years, as they come for medical help, and also the Indians as from time to time the colonist leaders advise them.

He was also "to educate and instruct in his art one or two youths fit to learn that profession, who if occasion serve, could succeed him in the Plantation."[4] There seems to be no record as to whether he did so.

Samuel Fuller, a London physician, came to Plymouth with William Bradford in 1620 and served not only the *Mayflower* passengers for the thirteen years he had yet to live, but also those who called for help in Boston and neighboring settlements. After his death in 1633 (from smallpox), his widow was allowed to keep an apprentice to continue his work. She was one of the several trained midwives in this early settlement. Boston, as well as most other early towns, also had a resident midwife. A few towns even had a resident physician. Richard Palgrave, from Stepney, Middlesex, was the first medical man in Charlestown, where he served the community for twenty years. Dr. Simon Eire came early to Watertown and stayed ten years. John Sprague, who followed John Clark to Newbury, stayed for forty-seven years.

Traditions cluster around the name of John Clark (1598–1664), surgeon and first physician of Newbury, and the progenitor of a family of seven physicians. Presumably with formal training behind him, according to Thacher's *Medical Biography,* Clark had been honored with a diploma for his "success in cutting for the Stone." On September 28, 1638, the town of Newbury "in respect of his calling, made him free from all public rates either for town or county so long as he remain and exercise his calling among us."[5] In 1652 the General Court awarded him a patent "for inventing a stove that saved firewood admirably." Doubtless Benjamin Franklin knew about this achievement. Dr. Clark also owned a large farm in Plymouth where he bred fine horses and cattle.

Hawthorne's choice of him as the physician in his romantic tales of the Province House a hundred years later recalled his name and helped to give it an even longer memory. In the tale of "Eleanora's Mantle," the story of an early smallpox outbreak in Boston, it is Dr. Clark who diagnoses the malady of the proud Eleanora as smallpox, during the Governor's reception for her at Province House. With all of socially important Boston present at this gala affair and the ball in full swing, Dr. Clark, who has been intently watching from the stair landing, calls the Governor aside and tells him what he has discovered. In a moment the Governor announces that the reception is ended, gaiety is over, and the puzzled guests depart. Dr. Clark attends the Lady Eleanora during the grim days that follow and watches her die.

A lithograph of Dr. Clark's portrait is the frontispiece of Joshua Coffin's *A Sketch of the History of Newbury,* and the original portrait, an oil painting owned by the Massachusetts Historical Society, now hangs in the Francis A. Countway Library of Medicine in Boston.

John Winthrop brought with him to Boston in 1630, on his flagship, the *Arbella,* Giles Firmin, an apothecary, with his son, a student in medicine at the University of Cambridge. The elder Giles Firmin died in 1634, and his son returned to England to complete his professional training. Having gained his degree, he returned to New England, accepted a pastorate in Ipswich, where he preached and practiced medicine until 1644 when he went back to England. Record of early medical service in the colonies, short or long, if collected, might change the medical story for these early years quite materially. Instead, we have only a few random names, unclothed with the details which might transform them into living individuals.

As the years went on from the 1702 outbreak to the arrival of the British ship *Seahorse* in 1721, smallpox memories of the first century grew dim and the present seemed to offer no threat. This interval of nineteen years was the longest since 1677, when the most severe outbreak of the first century had occurred.

IV

First Hope from Far Places

NEW ENGLAND'S FIRST hope of preventing smallpox infection appears to have come not from a physician directly or in print. Instead, it came from the mouth of an African slave, newcomer to the household of Cotton Mather, pastor of the North Church in Boston. From Mather's diary, under date of December 15, 1706, we read that "Some gentlemen of our Church, understanding . . . that I wanted a good *Servant* at the expense of between forty and fifty Pounds, purchased for me, a very likely *Slave*, a young Man, who is a Negro of a promising Aspect and Temper, and this Day they presented him unto me. I putt upon him the Name of *Onesimus*."[1]

In natural consequence of this addition to a Boston household, the new master soon would ask the new servant, "Have you ever had the smallpox?" Cotton Mather asked this inevitable question, and in partial reply, Onesimus rolled up his sleeve and showed the smallpox scar on his upper arm. America's share in the successful conquest of smallpox began at precisely this minute.

Cotton Mather does not mention asking this question in his 1706 diary entry, but he recalls the interview ten years later in a letter to Dr. John Woodward of the Royal Society in London. The date of this letter is July 12, 1716, and the occasion was Mather's reply to Dr. Woodward's letter concerning Mather's contribution of *Curiosa Americana* (second series), excerpts from which had been printed in the spring issue of the *Philosophical Transactions*, official organ of the Society for that year. Apparently Dr. Woodward had commented favorably about an article on inoculating for smallpox that had been printed in the same issue of the *Transactions*.[2] Mather's recall of the Onesimus interview in this connection is important enough to Boston's smallpox story to be reported in his own words from this 1716 letter. He wrote:

> I am willing to confirm you, in a favorable opinion, of Dr. Timonius's Communication; and therefore, I do assure you, that many months before I mett with any Intimations of treating ye Small-Pox with ye Method of Inoculation, I had from a Servant of my own, an Account of its being practiced in *Africa.* Enquiring of my Negro-Man *Onesimus,* who is a pretty Intelligent Fellow, Whether he ever had ye Small-Pox, he answered *Yes* and *No;* and then told me that he had undergone an Operation, which had given him something of ye Small-Pox, and would forever preserve him from it, adding, That it was often used among y^e *Guaramantese,* and whoever had ye Courage to use it, was forever free from ye Fear of the Contagion. He described ye Operation to me, and showed me in his Arm ye Scar, and his description of it made it the same that afterwards I found related unto you by your Timonius.[3]

This was Dr. Emanuel Timonius, doctor of medicine from the Universities of Oxford and Padua, now in Constantinople, who in 1713 had sent Dr. Woodward a letter telling of inoculation which he had known about for eight years and had witnessed in Constantinople. Dr. Woodward had translated the letter into English and had printed it in the *Philosophical Transactions* of the Royal Society in the spring issue for 1714. This English translation made the fact of inoculation available to English-speaking readers, as an earlier mention of it in Leipzig had failed to do.

In the letter to which Cotton Mather was replying on July 12, 1716, this favorable opinion of inoculation confirmed his own view of the Timonius letter. He does not say when he had read it. Dr. William Douglass, a Boston physician, who later lent Mather the Royal Society volume containing the letter, arrived in Boston in 1715 but became a permanent resident only after 1718. In 1716 when Mather was replying to Dr. Woodward, he had not yet heard of Dr. Jacob Pylarinus, another witness to inoculation, whose testimony to its effectiveness was also printed in the *Philosophical Transactions*.[4] Both of these physicians were replying to the Society's request for eyewitness accounts of the marvels of nature in all corners of the world.

Cotton Mather's *Curiosa Americana* was in answer to this same request. Each of the three series of examples he sent to Dr. Woodward contained widely varied examples of the following such marvels: a fossil tooth, a plant that cured rattlesnake bites, another that cured the *King's Evil,* wild turkeys weighing fifty or sixty pounds, flights of pigeons probably bound to some distant planet, monstrous births, medicines revealed in dreams, the Indian way of counting time by sleeps, moons, winters, uncommon rainbows and mock suns, a murder revealed in a dream, long-lived persons. Interest in both England and America was keenly awake to these teasing mysteries.[5]

Previously marvels of this unproved sort had been usually regarded as Providences of God for which no explanation was necessary. Cotton Mather had begun to help his father, Increase Mather, compile such a list until, perhaps unconsciously in response to a new time spirit, he was transferring his choices to nature. The *Curiosa Americana* shows something of this shift. In addition to the fact that he knew a little about smallpox from his own case as a fifteen-year-old boy, as well as from the anxiety of the 1702 outbreak that affected his family severely, he had for a time looked forward to a medical career himself and read medicine as a beginning toward that end. This was during the early period when his persistent habit of stammering threatened to make a pulpit career impossible. He conquered the stammering, however, and the pulpit won after all. Although the interest in medicine continued to the end of his life, he was simply a sharp observer, always a complete layman looking in from the outside.

The Timonius article was a careful physician's description of an unlikely phenomenon for which the author offered no guarantee, claimed no proofs, and made no recommendations. Through his eight years in Turkey, he had heard of no deaths from it nor of anyone who suffered from smallpox after inoculation, but his plainspoken article went no further. Cotton Mather accepted his story as completely authoritative, stating later that he was as certain that inoculation was safe and effective in creating immunity as he was that there are lions in Africa. One might observe that his grounds for believing in the lions were hardly impregnable. His positiveness is amazing, but it need not rob him of the distinction which fairly enough belongs to him for various reasons, among them his imaginative suggestion that contagion might arise from the existence of the "animated particles" the "glass" revealed in the smallpox pustule.[6] To the last line of his thousand pages in favor of inoculation, Cotton Mather never doubted the blessing of this discovery to the human race.

What Timonius and Pylarinus had done by putting their observations in print had opened the door to doubt and skepticism and to the incentive for further investigations which otherwise alert men would pursue. The first chapter in the long and bitter struggle toward further knowledge which Cotton Mather's confidence had triggered would take place in colonial Boston, beginning in 1721, but it would take the greater part of a full century before other men would find the way to discover a safer preventive to smallpox infection and then nearly two more centuries to eradicate the scourge from the earth.

As a folk custom inoculation had been practiced for centuries in China, India, and other Asiatic countries, as well as in Africa among primitive tribes. Through many generations, perhaps centuries, inoculation had remained within the realm of the folk practice, no doubt observed by travelers among similarly primitive groups that were widely separated and unable to communicate with each other. Carried to Europe perhaps as early as the sixteenth century, its procedures were still identical with those of these primitive tribes, presumably much earlier.

Descriptions of the disease of smallpox occur very early. That of Rhazes, remembered as the greatest physician of the ninth century in the Islamic world (c. A.D. 865–923/932), was the first to describe the disease with precise accuracy — particularly in discriminating between smallpox and measles, so often confused in later times. Rhazes is apparently the first writer to attempt so thorough an account of smallpox. His knowledge seems to have come from Aaron, a native of Alexandria, who lived about A.D. 622. (Smallpox having appeared in Arabia as early as A.D. 572, Mohammed's birth year.) A translation of the work of Rhazes from Greek into Latin by Nicholaus Machellus and printed in 1555 is said to have been the tenth edition of his work in print. By the eighteenth century various English translations were available, but comparison between these translations shows considerable variation in the text, as is understandable considering the number of earlier editions.[7]

Another reason for the importance of Cotton Mather's letter in 1716 to Dr. Woodward of the Royal Society is that it registers his intention to call a consultation of Boston doctors on inoculation, if smallpox came again to the town. His assumption that these men were ignorant of the letters of Timonius and Pylarinus was perhaps mistaken, but be that as it may, it was his letter to them that precipitated the bitter quarrel over inoculation in Boston and divided the town into hostile camps for many months. The significance of this quarrel when viewed at long range is that it led to a better way of dealing with smallpox and for that reason is still remembered.

Toward the end of the letter, Cotton Mather wrote, "For my own part, if I should live to see y^e *Small-Pox* again enter o'r City, I should immediately procure a Consult of o'r Physicians to introduce a Practice, which may be of so very happy a Tendency."[8]

This stated purpose appears in almost the same words in Mather's diary on May 26, 1721, when Boston was again in siege. The entry reads:

I will procure a Consult of our Physicians, and lay the matter before them.[9]

The letter is dated June 6, 1721.

V

One Practitioner
for Each Thousand Residents

COMPLETE AND ACCURATE information about Boston's medical protection at any given time in early years is hard to come by, and before the end of the first quarter of the eighteenth century, it is all but impossible. However, from such informal sources as are still available, it would seem that at this date there was at least one resident practitioner for each one thousand of the town's inhabitants. Unlike their earlier predecessors, these ten or eleven men were following one profession, not two or three; they had behind them an early apprenticeship followed by several years of practical experience instead of a university degree.

We have little more information about most of these men than such incidental items as found their way into newspapers, diary entries, letters, or other informal reports. Their medical records are lacking, and unless they published signed articles or pamphlets, extant materials are too scant from which to form a critical appraisal of their service. There were still a few pastor-physicians in Boston, as in small or remote country districts and possibly at least several English- or European-trained men who remained residents only briefly in the new world. Generally speaking, however, the remark of Dr. William Douglass, a three-year resident in 1721, fits the case.

"We abound in practitioners, but no other graduate than myself," he wrote in a letter to Cadwallader Colden, of New York Colony. Douglass never tired of reminding the "abounding practitioners" of his unique qualification and never quite accepted these fellow practitioners as colleagues. "Nevertheless," he added in the same letter, "I have resolved to fix here, and wander no more. I can live handsomely on the income of my practice here, and can save some small matter." He continued with comment which, disparaging as it may be, gives some hint of medical practice at this date, when conditions were normal. He wrote:

> I reckon this place at present no better than a factory, as to my interest, for here we have a great Trade and many Strangers with whom my business chiefly consists. I have Practice amongst four sorts of People: some families pay me five pounds per annum each for advice sick or well, some few fee me as in Britain, but for the native New Englanders I am obliged to keep a day book of my Consultations, Advice and Visits and bring them in a bill; others of the poorer sort I advise and visit without any expectation of fees.[1]

This letter was written immediately before the smallpox outbreak of 1721 that changed Boston life in nearly all directions for many months and tested each physician in new ways. It would be important to know the age of most Boston doctors at this date, for the young among them probably had never had a smallpox patient before, during the nineteen years of freedom from infection since 1702.

In comparison with still earlier times, medical experience at this date, due to the casualties in King Philip's War, included more experience in surgery than earlier generations had possessed. In 1675 young men who were looking forward to a medical career and had completed their apprenticeship, or nearly so, were assigned as assistants to army surgeons to be learners. It was a grim assignment, but it sorted out a few men with an aptitude for surgery, some of whom, after this introduction to the first principles and skills, went on with their training. Hitherto there had been very little specialized training for surgery.

The sharp distinction in England between physicians and surgeons had not been carried over to America. Nor were barber surgeons and apothecaries separate groups in Boston. At this time there were fourteen apothecary shops, each one owned and managed by a physician who collected, prepared, and handled his own medicines. He made his own powders, rolled his own pills, spread his own plasters, and supplied his patients with all medicines. Combining the professions of physician and apothecary, New England practitioners were spared the rivalry and jealousy English physicians had suffered from apothecaries for many years. Much mischief had resulted in the old country from apothecaries taking it upon themselves to prescribe as well as prepare drugs, and it was a long time before they learned either by trial and error, or later still, by getting the training offered to them in Scottish universities, to gain the confidence of the practitioners. New England not only had missed the confusion of this long process, but had also lacked the supervision and discipline of the College of Physicians.

The best known of the early teaching surgeons in New England was John Cutler, a Hollander, who first settled in Hingham and practiced there before King Philip's War. Best known by his Dutch name, De Messmaker, and popularly called "the Dutchman," he is listed in war records by his translated name, *Cutler,* which he kept after moving to Boston in 1694. He lived there for twenty-three years, attained wealth and eminence in his profession, and during these years trained young men in medicine and surgery. No better surgical training was available in New England during those years. Cutler died in 1717.[2] Had he lived but five years longer, his presence in Boston might have made a great difference in the bitter professional warfare of the tragic year 1721.

One of the young men who availed himself of Dr. Cutler's tutelage was Zabdiel Boylston, who is remembered primarily for what he accomplished during that fatal year of the siege. He was a third generation American, born March 6, 1669/1670. He was the son of Dr. Thomas Boylston, physician and surgeon in the village of Muddy River, now Brookline, and grandson of Thomas Boylston from London, one of the early settlers in Watertown. Zabdiel was the seventh of twelve children in his family, and the only one of six sons to follow his father's profession. No record of his early training is extant, but one might naturally suppose that during his early boyhood he had what amounted to a parental apprenticeship. His father died when Zabdiel was fifteen years old, and by that time he would have had at least two years of such training, more intimately conducted than it would have been in the home of a Boston master.

During his boyhood years, Muddy River was a sparsely settled area of near wilderness, five thousand acres and still tributary to Boston. There were less than three hundred residents by 1700, and a large portion of these picturesque acres was still almost untouched by cultivation. Boundaries marking the neighborhood settlements were indefinite. In all directions, this region was still more the haunt of beast rather than the dwelling place of man.

As a boy in these parts, Zabdiel Boylston lived a pioneer life closer to that of his grandfather, Thomas Boylston of London, than to that of his own father, Thomas Boylston, who had lived in Watertown before he moved to Muddy River after his father's death. As a boy Zabdiel Boylston looked out on rolling meadows, swamps thinly covered with water, densely wooded areas, small streams running back and forth between Muddy River and the Charles. It was a setting in which one's nearest neighbor was too far away for the light from his windows or the smoke from his chimney to be visible. No generation of boys born after 1700 would again grow up in such a paradise of adventure and discovery as the six boys of the Boylston household enjoyed during the last decade of the seventeenth century. Dr. Thomas Boylston's widely scattered patients demanded long horseback journeys through these thinly settled acres in all weathers, and stocking his own apothecary shop in season meant excursions through woods and fields and swamps in search of medicinal plants and their preparation at home for medicines he would need. As a physician in Boston, Zabdiel Boylston owned one of the largest apothecary shops of the town, and he had assembled a distinguished botanical collection. The beginnings of all this probably lay deep in his boyhood experience under the guidance and in the companionship of his father. The emphasis of Thomas Boylston's training might naturally have been surgical, as surgery was his own specialty after his service in King Philip's War.

Nothing is known of Zabdiel Boylston's association with John Cutler in Boston except that they seemed to have remained together for some time after Boylston's training period would have been completed. Boylston married in 1706 and took up residence in Dock Square where he established his practice and set up his apothecary shop as well.

Wilderness born, and, during his early years, wilderness bred, with excellent training and nearly fifteen years of independent medical practice behind him, Zabdiel Boylston was no longer a mere beginner in 1721. He belonged to New England and New England belonged to him — landscape, seasons, activities, people — and when his life was spent, he died in the house in which he was born. Life in the wilderness had instilled in him qualities of courage and independence that mark his story wherever some piece of it can still be uncovered.[3]

Who were his colleagues in Boston as the terrible year of 1721 approached? First, there was William Douglass, twelve years younger than Boylston and leader of the opposition against the use of inoculation. He was a man opposite to Boylston in most fundamental ways. Although Douglass chose New England as a place in which to practice medicine, he remained a Scot at heart, an alien in a foreign land. Formally educated in three English and European universities, and having received a degree from one of them, Douglass's academic career had brought him wide interests, standards of orderly procedure, a respect for fact, but an unfortunate blindness to the possibility of learning outside college halls. Not to have been formally educated was not to have been educated at all. However, life would teach him differently, to some degree. Later he had the honesty to record a change of mind as to inoculation and to use it in his practice, but to the last word he ever wrote he made not the slightest gesture of forgiveness to a colleague whom he had abused and deeply wronged for being successful on the other side of the public quarrel. He ignored and abused those whom he did not consider his peers, even attributing their success to ignoble motives.

His two essays on inoculation invited debate from those he opposed, but he gave them no chance. These essays have an historical importance. They clarify issues that had been befogged by lack of knowledge and postponement of experiment. They exhibit a step-by-step advance to a decision by a mind trained in accurate observation and willingness to be patient.[4]

Thomas Robie of Cambridge, a member of the Harvard College staff, a Fellow of the Royal Society, also took part in the 1721 inoculations and sent various reports of his observations to the Society. A few entries from his diary are extant. Thomas Bulfinch, who had been apprenticed to Zabdiel Boylston, left for Paris to complete his medical education and returned too late to take part in the 1721 experience or to accept Boylston's invitation to be his partner. Oliver Noyes, mentioned often by Samuel Sewall for his medical service, died in 1721, aged forty-eight. Doctors Cooke, Oakes, and Williams were also frequently mentioned in Sewall's diary as serving his family. Cotton Mather often spoke favorably of his neighbor, Dr. John Perkins. There was also Lawrence Dalhonde, formerly a physician in the French army, author of the frightening report on inoculation; and Dr. White, who supported Cotton Mather's letter to the Boston physicians; but even a full list of these incidental references to members of the profession in Boston at this time illuminates the situation very slightly. Boston's resource for active service during a period of desperate need remained within the skill and endurance of ten or twelve men to care for the probable six thousand who would need them.

VI

Boston's Great Plague Year, 1721

ON APRIL 22, 1721, the Boston *Gazette* reported in the issue of April 17 to 24, that "on Saturday last arrived here, His Majesty's ship, *Seahorse,* and several other ships from Saltertuda." The usual procedure as to illness on board had apparently been answered in the negative at the three-mile point before the ship proceeded to the dock. The company on board were on cruise and a brief pause was intended, but before the ship sailed again, word came that a Negro on board "sick with the smallpox" had been taken to a house near the shore. The selectmen immediately furnished a nurse to care for him, with orders not to leave the house without direction from this body. A red flag reading "God have mercy on this house" was raised at the door, and "two prudent persons" were sent to stand guard, allowing no one to enter or depart. This was routine procedure.

Several days later word came that another Negro on the ship, servant to Captain Wentworth Paxson, had been taken to the captain's house, also near the shore, "sick with the smallpox." The selectmen's orders were repeated. On this same day, John Clark was "desired by the Selectmen to go on board and Report back what state of Health or Sickness the Ship's Company was in." Apparently this May 8 report was favorable, but on May 22 the ship was ordered to proceed to Bird Island. While a pilot was being secured, but before the ship sailed, word came that more men of the crew were sick and that only ten or twelve men were left to handle the ship. Also on May 22 the *Boston News Letter* announced that "eight men and no more" were sick with the smallpox. On May 24 the selectmen ordered the twenty-six free Negroes in town to clean the streets. This also was a routine precaution, which after a full month's time would have carried small comfort to the knowing.

On May 26 Cotton Mather wrote in his diary, "The grievous calamity of the smallpox has now entered the town." It was even so. Day after day the number of cases increased. The selectmen continued the routine orders, finding nurses, appointing guards, raising red flags at the doors of infected houses. Scores of residents, especially those with young children, left town immediately if some family connection who lived reasonably close to town would take them in, for already it was recognized that infection from smallpox was by direct contact alone and distance meant safety. Perhaps of Boston's 11,000 residents at this date, as many as a thousand found such protection elsewhere. Perhaps also an approximate half of the adult population possessed immunity from the outbreaks of 1689–1690 and 1702, and of the older fraction a few from the severe siege of 1677. No child, however, born during the last nineteen years had a chance of safety.

These same nineteen years of freedom from smallpox fears meant for a large proportion of the total adult population scant familiarity with the many precautions, safeguards, and responsibilities which a major crisis imposed upon young or old. All were unready, and it would take time to learn caution afresh. The most disastrous outbreaks were always those after a long period of safety, and that 1721 would be a fatal year might easily have been predicted after the public announcement that eight men and no more were "sick with the smallpox." As early as May 26 when Cotton Mather made the entry in his diary, it was still too early for anyone to predict that this year's story would also bring the beginning of new hope for the future.

Mather's entry continues in these words:

The Practice of conveying and suffering the Small-Pox by Inoculation, has never been used in *America,* nor indeed in our

Nation, but how many Lives might be saved by it, if it were practiced. I will procure a Council of our Physicians, and lay the Matter before them.[1]

He had waited five years for this chance, since, in his letter to Dr. Woodward of the Royal Society dated July 12, 1716, he had first delivered this purpose to call a council in case smallpox came again to Boston. The words of the letter and those of the May 26 diary entry are identical. How heavily this purpose had rested in his mind one may only surmise, but at least he had not forgotten his intent on the very day it was needed. More important still, the writing of the letter to the Boston doctors, detailing his small knowledge of inoculation, was not born of a sudden impulse but was considered action with a long stretch of time behind it.

He sent his summons to the doctors on June 6 and recorded it in his diary: "I write a Letter to the Physicians, entreating them to take into consideration the important Affair of preventing the *Small Pox* in the way of Inoculation." Since the beginning of the outbreak a month before, he had borrowed from Dr. Douglass the Royal Society volume containing the Timonius article and the later abstract of the Pylarinus article translated by Dr. Woodward. He quotes from both of these in his letter without mentioning Dr. Douglass or making acknowledgment to him. How many of Boston's physicians were summoned to this *Consult,* who they were, or how the letter was received is unknown. We know only that no *Consult* was held, and that Dr. White alone was said to have expressed good will.

The letter as a whole has never been printed and was apparently in a single copy, passed from hand to hand among the physicians. As to the precise text, we have only Mather's diary entries and in Chapter XX of *The Angel of Bethesda* what was probably close to the original version of what he had written. The conclusion of the letter, as there recorded, reads:

Gentlemen, my request is, that you meet for a Consultation
upon this occasion, and deliberate upon it (the operation) that
whosoever first begins the practice (if you approve it should be
done at all) may have the countenance of his worthy Brethren
to fortify him in it.[2]

Quite definitely he did not urge the inoculation, but only deliberation
on it and action as a unit if they approved it should be attempted
at all. His own diary word *entreat* is stronger than his letter.

What Cotton Mather was incapable of realizing was that as a
self-appointed representative, appealing to a group of men of another profession, he was not likely to be welcomed or his suggestion
heeded. He crossed all such boundaries without a scruple and with
no sense of impropriety or discourtesy. On one earlier occasion he
had written in his diary, "Our excellent Governour is in danger of
some Steps inconvenient for himself and us. No body will advise
him. I must."[3] The sense of authority came in part from being the
son of Increase and the grandson of Richard Mather from whom
he had inherited, despite all contradiction, the notion of ministerial
privilege and duty. This is a front-line clue to the understanding of
Cotton Mather's behavior in every chapter of his life. As to his
own deep concern for Boston's welfare in the 1721 crisis, there is
not the shadow of a doubt. He cared, and the *must* was upon him;
therefore he acted, time after time, without tact or consideration.
Whether the situation resulting from his letter to the physicians or
the immediate demand of Dr. Douglass for the return of the volume,
from which citations were made without acknowledgment, suggested to Cotton Mather that he had made a mistake in so doing is
not known. Dr. Douglass demanded the return of the book and
refused to lend it again, even to the Governor, whose interest in the
inoculation accounts at this moment of Boston's anxiety needs no
explanation.

The next day, June 24, Mather wrote also to Zabdiel Boylston, one of Boston's ten physicians, his neighbor, and apparently a close acquaintance. This letter has almost an intimate tone, uncommon in Mather's correspondence. He wrote:

> You are many ways, Sir, endeared unto me, but in nothing more than in the very much good which a gratious God employs you and honours you in a miserable world.
>
> I design it, as a testimony and esteem that I now lay before you, the most that I know (and all that was ever published in the world) concerning a matter, which I have the occasion of its being much talked about. If upon mature deliberation, you should think it admissable to be proceeded in, it may save many lives that we set a great store on. But if it be not approved of, you will have the pleasure of knowing what is done in other places. . . .
>
> But now think, Judge, do as the Lord our healer shall direct you, and pardon the freedom of
>
> Sir, Your hearty friend and Servant,
co. Mather.[4]

As in his letter to the town physicians the day before, Cotton Mather puts Boylston under no pressure to act, but according to Boylston's own statement years later, it was this letter that sparked his decision. He wrote of it, "Upon reading of which I was very well pleas'd, and resolv'd in my Mind to try the Experiment." He did so two days later, June 26.

Boylston could not inoculate himself, since he had acquired the immunity of a survivor in the outbreak of 1702. Accordingly, he chose his six-year-old son, who had not gone with his mother when she left town with the other young children at the beginning of the outbreak. He also inoculated one of his slaves, Jack, aged thirty-six, and Jack's two-and-a-half-year-old son, Jacky.

Before sunset of this June 26 day, all of Boston knew what Boyl-

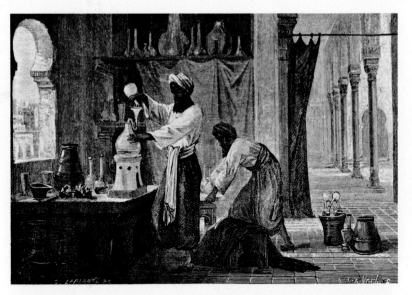

Rhazes in his laboratory, included without mention of artist or source in *Vies des Servants du Moyen Age* by Louis Figuier, Paris, 1867. Rhazes (Abu-Bakr Mohammed Ibu Zakariya Al Razi) c. 852–932, Arab physician, author of *A Treatise on Small Pox and Measles*, perhaps the earliest accurate description of smallpox in print.

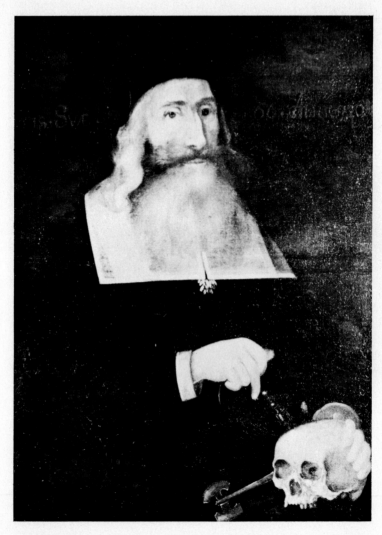

John Clark, 1598–1664, resident of Newbury and one of the earliest trained physicians of the Massachusetts Bay Colony. His portrait is attributed to Augustine Clement. (Courtesy of the Boston Medical Library in the Francis A. Countway Library of Medicine.)

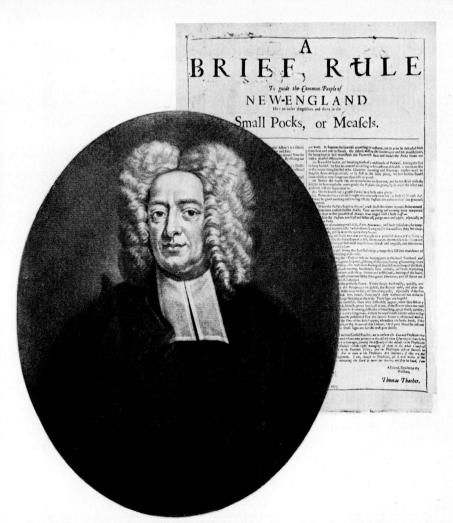

Broadside by Thomas Thacher, *A Brief Rule To guide the Common-People of New-England How to order themselves and theirs in the Small Pocks, or Measels*, Boston, 1677. (Courtesy of the Boston Public Library.)

Cotton Mather, 1663–1728, Boston clergyman and writer, pastor of the North Church, initial advocate of inoculation in the smallpox epidemic of 1721, and active participant in the bitter controversy that followed. Portrait by Peter Pelham. (Courtesy of the Boston Athenaeum.)

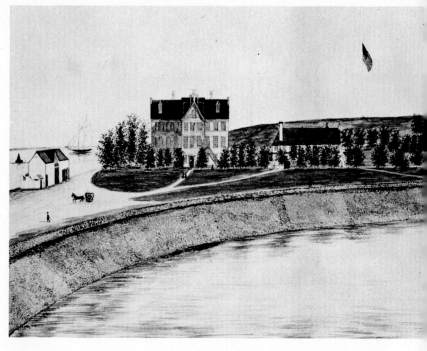

Boston's first Quarantine Hospital, originally set up on Spectacle Island in 1717, moved to Rainsford Island in 1737, continued as a quarantine hospital until 1849, when it became a poorhouse. The wash painting, by an unknown artist, was made in 1865. (Courtesy of the Boston Medical Library in the Francis A. Countway Library of Medicine.)

Opposite: Title page of Zabdiel Boylston's *An Historical Account of the Small-Pox Inoculated in New England*, London, 1726. (Courtesy of the Francis A. Countway Library of Medicine.) Below: Zabdiel Boylston's signature. (Courtesy of the British Museum.)

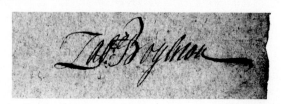

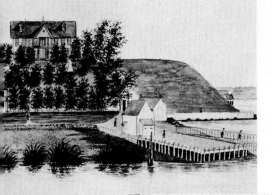

AN

Hiſtorical ACCOUNT

OF THE

SMALL-POX

INOCULATED

IN

NEW ENGLAND,

Upon all Sorts of Perſons, *Whites, Blacks,*
and of all Ages and Conſtitutions.

With ſome Account of the Nature of the
Infection in the NATURAL and INOCULATED
Way, and their different Effects on HUMAN
BODIES.

With ſome ſhort DIRECTIONS to the UN-
EXPERIENCED in this Method of Practice.

Humbly dedicated to her Royal Highneſs the Princeſs of WALES,
By *Zabdiel Boylſton*, F. R. S.

The Second Edition, Corrected.

LONDON:

Printed for S. CHANDLER, at the Croſs-Keys in the *Poultry.*
M. DCC. XXVI.

Re-Printed at *BOSTON* in *N. E.* for S. GERRISH in
Cornhil, and T. HANCOCK at the Bible and Three Crowns
in *Annſtreet.* M. DCC. XXX.

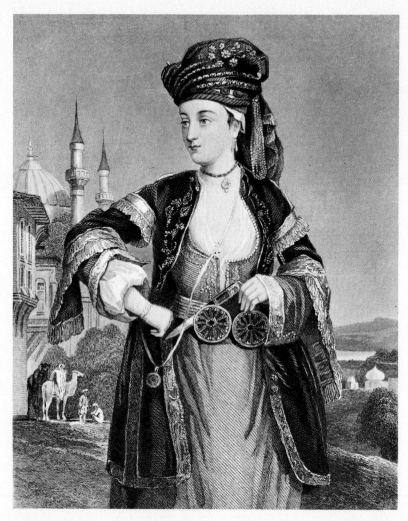

Lady Mary Wortley Montagu, 1689–1762, famous English letter
writer, who in 1721, having had her son and daughter inoculated, took
a brief share in the English attempt to convince the public that inoculation was a safe and effective protection against smallpox infection. Portrait by J. B. Wanderforde, engraved by S. Hollyer. (Courtesy of the
Boston Athenaeum.)

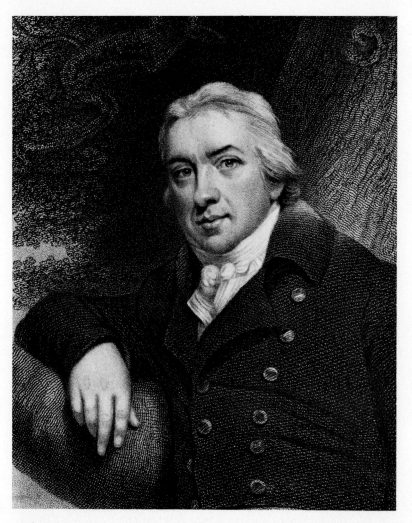

Edward Jenner, 1749–1823, physician of Gloucestershire, England, who developed the idea of vaccination with cowpox virus to replace the former folk practice of direct inoculation from the smallpox pustule. Engraved by J. R. Smith. (Courtesy of the Boston Athenaeum.)

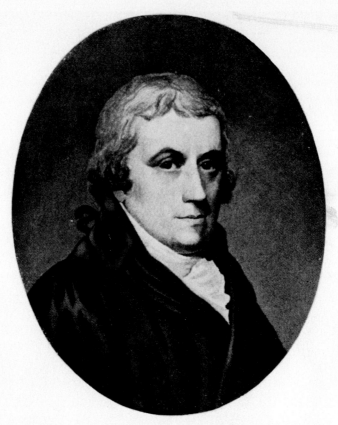

Benjamin Waterhouse, 1754–1846, Boston physician and professor of the Theory and Practice of Physic at Harvard College, who planned and carried through a public experiment to demonstrate the safety and effectiveness of Jennerian vaccination with cowpox virus, Boston, 1802. Engraved by S. Harris. (Courtesy of the Boston Athenaeum.)

ston had done, as the new word *inoculation* traveled up and down every street, explaining nothing to the uninitiate. The first response, naturally enough, was a sense of complete shock. Dr. Boylston, known to many residents as a friend and helpful physician through fifteen years, had inoculated his own child. How could he, and what would this new fear mean to Boston already terrified, as infection spread and new cases were reported by the hour? The sense of shock increased as news came that all the other doctors of the town were solidly against Dr. Boylston's use of inoculation, which was insufficiently tested and also possibly highly dangerous. There is scant reason to assume that their opposition was born either of undue ignorance, or of malice toward Dr. Boylston, who, as they thought, was acting in too great haste and with indiscretion.

The tumult of the people is no puzzle. It was born of fear, which as the cases increased and the first deaths were announced, mounted to terror. Cotton Mather wrote it down as "clamour," wild clamor. The devil himself had taken possession of the people. "They rave, they rail, they blaspheme; they talk not only like Ideots, but also like *Fanaticks,* and not only the Physician who began the Experiment, but I also am the subject of their Fury; their furious Obliquies and Invectives."[5] Day by day Mather's superlatives as to the violence of this uproar increased until Boston itself had become almost "an hell on earth." One may dismiss this extravagance as part of Mather's own idiom in the privacy of a diary page. He was conscious, no doubt, that he was not speaking for the whole of Boston, which was acting calmly. On June 22 the *Boston News Letter* announced that the Harvard commencement, which always brought large numbers from towns far and near, would be privately managed this year to avoid spreading contagion. On July 6 the foreign section of the paper, always the larger half, carried an article on the nature of contagion. In the following week there was an article by Dr. Mead, a London physician, on nursing the sick. In July 13 the proclamation of a Day of Humiliation throughout the Province appeared, "On

Occasion of the Calamity now upon miserable Boston." There was
no hysterical comment and no local mention of increasing cases.

The first public note of professional opposition to Boylston came
on July 21 in a meeting called by the selectmen. All of Boston's
physicians were present, as well as justices of the peace and other
officials, together with a considerable number of private citizens. The
purpose of the meeting was to hear a report prepared by Dr. Lawrence Dalhonde on the long-range effects of inoculation, as he had
allegedly observed them during his previous service in the French
army. Before the report was read, Dr. William Douglass asserted
under oath that the text of this report had been accurately translated into English. Nothing was said as to the accuracy of the report
itself, only of the translation.

The report reviewed the cases in three Instances:

> Instance 1. Of thirteen soldiers inoculated twenty-five years
> before in Cremona, four had died, six had suffered from paro-
> tidal tumors and a large inflammation in the throat, and three
> had been entirely unaffected.
>
> Instance 2. Of two soldiers inoculated twenty years before,
> one had been seized with ulcers of which he had died; the other
> had not been affected.
>
> Instance 3. Of two soldiers at the battle of Almanza in Spain,
> one had been unaffected, but the other, who had recovered from
> the inoculation, had been seized with a frenzy six weeks later
> and had died.[6]

In a calm moment years later, Zabdiel Boylston, recalling this
report, remarked that it was as likely of belief from the "knowing
Part of Mankind as if Dr. Dalhonde had said that the soldiers' heads
had fallen off or that the inoculation had changed men into women
or any other strange thought that might have come into his head."
On this July 21 occasion, however, the report was followed by a

resolution from the opposing physicians, that having discussed the report, they had concluded that "the Operation of Inoculation in Boston was likely to prove of dangerous consequence."

Given an opportunity to speak, Dr. Boylston stated that at the time he had seven patients under inoculation. He invited the physicians present to visit these patients and judge for themselves concerning their condition. No one accepted the invitation. The selectmen concurred with the opposing physicians and their report was ordered published.

As news of this meeting, of the Instances, the Resolution of the opposing physicians, and of Dr. Boylston's seven more inoculations was carried to every corner of Boston, public indignation, or what Cotton Mather called "frenzy" of the people, merely increased. Reasonable judgment had no chance. Boston had become a "dismal Picture and Emblem of Hell; Fire and Darkness filling of it and a Lying Spirit reigning there." The infection was spreading ever more rapidly, and another Mather diary item, "Widows multiply," was beginning to be almost literally true.

Three days after the Dalhonde episode, Dr. William Douglass, using the pseudonym William Philanthropos, which deceived no one, inserted a communication in the *Boston News Letter* in which he not only protested against inoculation, but also attacked Dr. Boylston personally in an abusive and insulting manner. He identified him as "a certain cutter for the Stone" — one of Dr. Boylston's especially successful operations — called him not only ignorant, but illiterate and incapable of understanding the writings of Timonius and Pylarinus, whose operation he had tried to copy. He was unacquainted with the treatment for smallpox, negligent in "not preparing the Bodies of his Subjects, unfit to manage any of their Symptoms, and in Propagating the Infection in the most Publick Trading Place in the Town, [Dock Square where Boylston lived]. If it kills the Patient, the Operator will be indicted for Felony."

The unprofessional character of this personal attack on his re-

spected colleague, senior to Douglass in age and experience by some
twelve years, deserved no answer, but only to be buried and forgotten. The first effect of the Douglass letter had been five days of
complete silence on both sides of the inoculation controversy. But,
after the first five days, in the next issue of the *Boston News Letter,*
a straightforward reply, signed by six of Boston's leading clergymen,
set the town talking more openly.

> It was grief to us the Subscribers, among others of your friends
> in the Town, to see Dr. Boylston treated so unhandsomely in
> the Letter directed to you last Week and Published in your
> Paper. He is a Son of the Town whom Heaven (as we all
> know) has adorned with some very peculiar Gifts for Service
> to his Country, and hath signally own'd in the Successes he has
> had.

Then follows a statement of Boylston's worth to Boston and to
the country, which by its positive tone and dignity put to shame the
malicious attack of Dr. Douglass. Wisely the six ministers, Increase
and Cotton Mather, Thomas Prince, William Cooper, and Benjamin
Colman — signers to the letter — offered no arguments in favor of
inoculation. They lacked the knowledge out of which arguments
might have come and knew that they lacked it, but they believed in
the integrity and good sense of Dr. Boylston. Their confidence in him
was not only inspiriting, but it also helped the cause with men of
judgment and politeness. Even as early as this in the controversy,
Boston ministers as a group would not only have been on Boylston's
side personally, but also would have favored inoculation.

Meanwhile clamor, rage, and insult went on as cases increased
and more deaths were reported day after day. Selectmen were as
busy as the doctors. Stricter quarantine was ordered against incoming ships, a house-to-house canvass was made to determine exactly
how many were ill. Meetings of the General Court were prorogued.

The Day of Humiliation and Fasting was observed. Zabdiel Boylston quietly resumed his inoculations.

His own statement in *Some Account of Inoculating or Transplanting the Small Pox and of the Benefit and Safety of the Practice* should have quieted the excitement of such abuse and unkindness as were being leveled against him, as well as revealing something significant as to Boylston's own spirit.

He wrote:

It might be easy for me to make answers to the Scurrilous things lately published against me, and satisfy the Publick of the Falsehood and Baseness in them, but I think it better becomes a considerate man to decline foolish Contentions particularly at a time when there is a *grievous Calamity* upon us, that calls us (instead of railing at one another) to unite in prayers to God for his Mercies to us. And therefore if any think to go on with their Calumnies and Fooleries I shall not think to take any notice of them. What I do (I hope as it has hitherto done) will vindicate itself with People of Thought and Probity.[7]

This was the treatise Cotton Mather had spoken of in his diary when he wrote, "I will allow the persecuted Physician to publish my Communications with the Levant, about the Small-Pox and supply him with further Ammunition to conquer the Dragon." On the title page of this piece Boylston called himself the publisher, not the author, which was to a degree correct. It is easy to separate the Mather and Boylston portions of this treatise. Mather keeps to the text of the Timonius letter; Boylston's comments stem from his own experience with his patients.

Boston was in no mood, however, to read about Timonius and Pylarinus or to make a reasonable judgment on the Dalhonde report. Dr. Boylston's seven more inoculations was the detail to be emphasized and magnified with each recital. Boston had almost truly become, in Mather's words, "a dismal Picture and Emblem of Hell; Fire and Darkness filling of it, and a lying spirit reigning there." At about this time Mather's son Samuel came home from Harvard terrified, for his chambermate had died of smallpox. Samuel begged to be inoculated, but his father hesitated. If he refused and then Sammy should die of the disease . . . "How can I answer it? If on the other Side, Our People, who have Satan filling their Hearts and their Tongues, will go on with infinite Prejudices against me and my ministry, If I suffer this Operation upon this Child, and be sure, if he should happen to miscarry under it, my Condition would be insupportable."

"Have it done privately," wise Grandfather Increase advised. This was done, and though Samuel's case went somewhat irregularly at first, after he had "a vein breathed in him," he improved and was presently well, and his worried father did not suffer "the prodigious Clamour and Hatred from an infuriated Mob, whom the Devil has inspired with a hellish rage, on this Occasion."

As July ended and August began, the severity of this epidemic increased with terror in proportion as the disease mounted to its usual peak in the months of September, October, and November. Whole families were laid low at the same time. More and more deaths were reported by the day. Funeral bells tolled all day long. Many shops were closed and business was almost at a complete standstill. Streets were deserted except for groups of mourners on their way to a funeral at one of the meetinghouses or waiting at the entrance to hold a service. At night the "dead cart" rumbled over the cobbled streets.

Boston's doctors had no rest day or night. With hundreds sick there were always calls that could not be answered. Selectmen were as busy as the doctors, week by week making themselves available day or night. The General Court was prorogued three times during this period. Their alternate meetingplace in early summer had been

Cambridge, which was now also under siege. Selectmen's orders give hints of problems that arose. In late July complaints against the continual ringing of funeral bells had led to an order that only one bell might be tolled at a time and that only at designated hours. A forty-shilling fine was imposed for disobedience to this order, but very soon it had to be rescinded. Boston's accustomed funeral pattern made obedience too painful to endure, and the bells rang again.

In September the sloop men refused to bring their loads of firewood as far as the dock for fear of infection. The selectmen met this difficulty by ordering that sloops be unloaded at Castle Island. The wood owners paid the price of unloading and the town met the charge of shuttle boats to the dock. Officers of military companies accustomed to drilling their men once a week were ordered not to call them forth in the time of public illness.

Sunday worship, however, was in no way restricted during all this long period of danger from infection. The understanding of contagion and quarantine went no further than the confining of those who were actually ill. Members of the family not yet ill occupied the family pew as usual, and as the deacon went up and down the aisle, they handed him the "Bills" requesting prayers for those ill at home. For several Sundays Cotton Mather noted the number of such requests at the North Church. On the "last Lord's Day," October 7, there were two hundred and two "Bills"; on October 14, three hundred and twenty-two "Bills." It is not surprising that the note added to these totals is "My Prayers for the Sick of the Flock now take up a very great deal of my Time."

In early October the selectmen ordered a house-to-house canvass to ascertain precisely how many had suffered the disease and how many had escaped. The number of workers required for the canvass, the fact that totals changed daily, the labor of keeping the records, and the difficulty of finding substitutes as sickness claimed members of any staff day after day, make the records as preserved something of an achievement.

On November 13 anger and bad feeling toward Cotton Mather found an ugly climax in the hurling of a homemade "granado" into his sleepingroom at 3:00 A.M. "By the Providence of God," however, as the local press reported this murderous purpose, as the heavy contrivance went through the window, the lighted fuse hit against the leaden frame and fell off, preventing an explosion, and possibly also the burning of Mather's house. By God's Providence also, Cotton Mather was not occupying his room on that night but had given it to his nephew, Thomas Walter, minister at Roxbury, who was recovering from inoculation. Wrapped around the "granado" was a blasphemous note, also preserved from burning, which indicated that a personal grudge against Mather from someone in his church was back of this wicked intent, not indignation due to his promotion of inoculation. For a time, as Mather confided to his diary, he was filled "with unutterable joy" at the thought of his approaching martyrdom when a second attempt, promised in the note, would "do the business" without fail. This attempt, however, did not materialize.

Boston was, of course, deeply shocked by this sensational affair. Governor Shute issued a proclamation on the following morning, offering a fifty-pound reward for any information as to the identity of the would-be murderer and immunity for any accomplice who would come forward with a clue, but no response came. Cotton Mather was already suffering considerable loss of ministerial prestige locally, because of his repeated criticism of James Franklin's new sheet, the *New England Courant,* which had very quickly assumed the role of an anti-inoculation newspaper in spite of occasionally printing an article favoring it to offset this impression. The "vile Courant" was Mather's phrase, and its spokesmen, direct agents of Satan. By calling names as his opponents were doing, he had allowed his side of the public quarrel to descend to a personal level, profiting nothing. Had he chosen silence, he would have been far wiser.

While the "granado" throwing was taking the center of the Boston stage, the selectmen were extending their house-to-house, street-by-street investigation to discover outsiders who were in town undergoing inoculation. Roxbury was one of the chief offenders in this forbidden adventure. By order of October 20, that any such offender would be immediately removed to Spectacle Island, lest "by allowing this Practice the Town be made an Hospital for that which may prove worse than the Small-Pox which has already put so many into Mourning." By harboring Thomas Walter of Roxbury, Cotton Mather had invited reproof for disobedience to this order made three weeks previously.

Relaxation of severity in imposing penalties for such disobedience was owing no doubt to the fact that during the late months of this year, inoculation had been gaining some favor in Boston. Discussions about it were growing less theoretical. People were not reading over and over what Timonius and Pylarinus had said. They were asking only on question — does it work? — and then intently watching for evidence. For a few days those who had been inoculated were not seen on the street, but very shortly they were out again and apparently in health. At least for them, inoculation had worked just as their ministers had said it would. Gradually this reassuring evidence began to be passed around, although the stern opposition of the selectmen kept it safely under cover.

Gradually also during November and December residents who had fled the town in April and May began to come back. Closed stores began to open. The Governor issued the usual Thanksgiving Proclamation. At the North Church the "Bills" for pastoral prayers fell to fifty in early December. Boston life began to resume its accustomed rhythm once more. As winter weather eased in late December and then more rapidly after the January thaw, spread of the disease diminished, although many were still ill. In February and March, no deaths were reported. In April there were two; in May only one. On May 14 a report in Town Meeting stated that no one had contracted smallpox for fourteen days. Six who had been inoculated were removed to Spectacle Island to complete their recovery. At this meeting Dr. Boylston agreed to inoculate no more patients without the approval of authority. The siege was over.

It had been a costly year. Figures vary slightly in different reports as to how many had been ill, but there was agreement as to the number of deaths. The selectmen's investigation had shown 5980 infected. Dr. Douglass said 6000. The Sewall and Prince reports show a slight variation in the total number infected, but 844 deaths and the proportion of one death "in every six, or between that of six or seven" cases held for all.[8]

VII

England's Promoter of Inoculation Was a Titled Lady

ENGLAND'S NONPROFESSIONAL promoter of inoculation was an even more unlikley advocate than New England's Calvinistic clergyman. She was a titled lady, a reigning beauty and wit at court, Lady Mary Wortley Montagu, famous in later times for her engaging letters to persons of quality in eighteenth-century high life. As she herself put it, "I came young into the hurry of the world." Truly enough, and before her mid-twenties, she had begun to build for herself a reputation for intellectual acumen as well as for charm and beauty. Through a long life she continued to enrich this tradition as her paths of adventure widened.

Her concern with smallpox began in 1713 when her brother died of it. Two years later, when she was living in London, she also contracted the disease, recovered, but with her beauty sadly marred. Her face was deeply pitted, and she had lost her eyelashes. Dr. Garth, an eminent court physician, who had attended her, had given his oath that she would again be fair, but no. "False was his oath; my beauty is no more!" she wrote. Her misfortune, however, did not affect her position at court. She returned, took her place as before, and though she used her wit more sharply, sometimes maliciously, she soon won the sympathy even of her enemies and, very shortly, their admiration as well.

In 1718 her husband, Edward Wortley, was appointed Ambassador Extraordinary to the Court at Constantinople. Lady Mary, equipped with an impressive retinue, set forth to this new scene of conquest, taking with her her six-year-old son. Soon after her arrival in Constantinople, she gave birth to a daughter. The physician chosen by the ambassador to care for his family was Dr. Maitland, and the Embassy surgeon was Dr. Emanuel Timonius, whose account of the Turkish method of inoculation had been printed in the Royal Society's *Philosophical Transactions* in 1714. Lady Mary had missed seeing this article, but soon after arriving in Constantinople and hearing of inoculation, she determined to have the operation performed on her six-year-old son. It was a daring step to take entirely on her own responsibility, but she took it immediately in consultation with Dr. Maitland and in the absence of her husband. Both Dr. Maitland and Dr. Timonius were present at the operation and Dr. Maitland assisted. His account is enlightening as the word of an experienced physician who took part in it, along with "the old Greek woman Lady Mary had engaged to perform it." He wrote:

The Ambassador's ingenious Lady, who had been at some Pains to satisfy her Curiosity in this Matter, and had made some useful Observations on the Practice, was so thoroughly convinced of the safety of it that *she* resolved to submit her only son to it, a very hopeful Boy of about six Years of Age.

She first of all order'd me to find out a fit Subject to take the Matter from: and then sent for an old *Greek* woman who had practic'd this Way a great many Years. After a great deal of Trouble and Pains, I found a proper Subject, and then the good Woman went to Work; but so awkwardly by the shaking of her Hand, and put the Child to so much Torture with her blunt and rusty Needle, that I pitied his Cries, who had ever been of such Spirit and Courage, that hardly any Thing of Pain could make him cry before: and therefore I Inoculated the other Arm with my own Instrument, and with so little Pain to him, that he did not in the least complain of it.[1]

Thereafter all went as predicted. The boy was only slightly ill, "for a few hours only and a week later was reported to be past all manner of danger."

Lady Mary's letter to Sarah Chiswell of Nottingham before the operation also has illuminating details about what Lady Mary called "the set of old women who make it their business to perform this operation every Autumn, in the month of September, when the great Heat is abated." She wrote in part:

> People send to one another to know if any member of their family has a mind to have the smallpox. They make partys for this purpose, and when they are met (commonly fifteen or sixteen together) the old woman comes with a nut-shell full of the matter of the best sort of smallpox, and asks what vein you please to have open'd. She immediately rips that open that you offer to her with a large needle (which gives you no more pain than a common scratch) and puts into the vein as much venom as you can lye upon the head of her needle and after that binds up the little wound with a hollow bit of shell, and in this manner opens four or five veins. The Grecians have commonly the superstition of opening one in the Middle of the forehead, one on each arm, and one on the breast, to mark the sign of the cross: but this has a very ill Effect. All these wounds leaving little Scars, and is not done by those who are not superstitious, who choose to have them in the legs or that part of the arm that is conceal'd. The children or young patients play together all the rest of the day, and are in perfect health to the eighth; Then the fever begins to seize them and they keep their beds two days, very seldom three. They have very rarely above twenty or thirty in their faces, which seldom mark, and in eight days' time they are as well as before their illness. . . .

The French Ambassador says pleasantly that they take the smallpox here by way of diversion as they take the Waters in other Countries. There is no Example of one that has dyed in it, and you may believe I am well satisfy'd of the Safety of the Experiment since I intend to try it on my dear little Son.

Lady Mary concluded this letter by saying:

I am Patriot enough to take pains to bring this useful Invention into new fashion in England, and I shall not fail to write to some of our own Doctors about it, if I know any one of em that I thought had Virtue enough to destroy such a considerable branch of their Revenue for the good of Mankind. Perhaps if I live to return, I may, however, have courage to war with em.[2]

On March 23 she wrote to her husband:

The Boy was engrafted last Tuesday and is at this time singing and playing and very impatient for his supper . . . I cannot engraft the girl; her nurse has not had the Small Pox.

On April 1 she wrote again to her husband:

Your Son is as well as can be expected, and I hope past all manner of danger.[3]

Back in London, Lady Mary was as good as her word in her letter to Sarah Chiswell. In 1721 when smallpox was epidemic in London, as in Boston, she determined to have her daughter inoculated and sent for Dr. Maitland, who advised waiting for better weather. Lady Mary did not wish to wait, and the operation was performed at once. Three learned physicians of the Royal College were present and watched with Dr. Maitland through the recovery of Miss Wortley. The weekly newspapers printed articles on inoculation and some interest was awakened in the subject. More interest followed when Princess Caroline, impressed by the success of the operation on Miss Wortley, determined to have her children inoculated also. This prospect necessitated more elaborate preparation. Six prisoners, condemned to die, volunteered to act as test cases and were promised freedom if they survived. Five of them had a light case of smallpox, as was expected, and they were freed. The sixth, upon dimly remembering hearing that as a child he had suffered smallpox, was allowed to go free as well.

Princess Caroline, not entirely reassured by these advance cases, wished further trial, and accordingly all the orphan children of St. James's parish were also inoculated. All survived, and this success seeming sufficient proof, the Princess engaged Dr. Maitland to inoculate two of her daughters. The favor of royalty gave more publicity to the operation and for a short time, Lady Mary's word *fashionable* was almost true. Then two deaths from inoculation: one a servant in Lord Bathhurst's household, and the other, the two-and-a-half-year-old son of the Earl of Sunderland, caused violent, adverse opinion.

Then, on July 2, 1722, a sermon preached by Edmund Massey at St. Andrew's, Holborn, stopped the practice entirely for a long time Massey's sermon was entitled "A Sermon Against the Dangerous and Sinful Practice of Inoculation." He took Job as his protagonist, a man who had baffled the devil, endured loss of estate, bereavement of his children, and then suffered a noisome distemper, "which might be what is now conveyed to men by some such way as that of inoculation which is derived from the same part of the world as was Job's scene of action. But in all his malicious Designs the Devil was disappointed." Then the preacher considered for what reason diseases are sent into the world. Certainly, to test our faith and to punish us for our sins. Who is it that hath the power of inflicting diseases upon us? God Almighty, who sometimes gives man the power to heal diseases, but never the power to inflict them. God

reserves that right unto himself alone. Adventurous practitioners
are usurping that power. They are tempting God by relying upon
themselves.

"The fear of disease is a happy restraint to men. If men were
more healthy, 'tis a great chance they would be less righteous. Let
the Atheist and the scoffer inoculate. Their hope is in and for only
this life. Let us bless God for the Afflictions He sends upon us, and
grant us patience under them."[4] These arguments were repeated by
others of the higher clergy, as they joined the opposition. Opposed
physicians were skeptical of the protective power of inoculation and
scornful of a method belonging to ignorant women and practiced
upon the illiterate and superstitious. The patronage of the royal
family was a humiliation of the English nation. Dr. William Wagstaffe's spirited pamphlet urging physicians not to allow their profession of healing to be usurped by amateurs called for refutation as
did Edmund Massey's sermon, and refutation came.

Lady Mary's indignation was immediate and she stepped into the
battle before allowing tempers to cool. She wrote an essay entitled
"A Plain Account of the Inoculating of the Small Pox," signing herself A Turkey Merchant — a disguise that was not discovered for
two hundred years. This essay appeared in the *Flying Post or Post-
master* when the controversy over the Massey sermon was at its
height, was widely read, and strongly effective — possibly because
the Turkey Merchant pseudonym gave the impression of being authoritative. The editor had apparently toned down the sarcastic
thrusts at the Royal College of Physicians with that hope in mind.
The opening paragraph deserves quotation. Lady Mary had written:

> Out of compassion to the numbers abused and deluded by the
> knavery and ignorance of physicians, I am determined to give
> a true account of the manner of inoculating the smallpox as it
> is practiced in Constantinople with constant success, and with-
> out any ill consequence whatever. I sell no drugs, take no fees,

could I persuade people of the safety and reasonableness of this easy operation. 'Tis no way my interest (according to the usual acceptation of that word) to convince the world of their errors, that is, I shall get nothing by it but the private satisfaction of having done some good to mankind, and I know nobody that reckons that satisfaction any part of their interest.[5]

By this appeal, to the reasonable reader, Lady Mary helped to popularize the method at the same time Dr. Jurin of the Royal Society was establishing, through statistics, the safety of it. The number of patients increased immediately, and the effect of the Massey sermon was weakened at the outset.

In addition to the influence of her essay, Lady Mary's unsparing willingness to visit the sick and to answer questions as to the inoculation of her daughter, who often accompanied her on her visits, meant that she was so urgently sought by parents undecided as to whether to risk the inoculation of their children that for a time her own pattern of life was sadly changed, and as she wrote to her sister, she was "obliged to run into the country." Worldly wise woman that she was, however, and having shot her bolt, she retired gracefully from the noise of battle and returned into the gaiety and tinsel glitter of court life which was her world.

VIII

Zabdiel Boylston in London

By MIDSUMMER, 1722, tempers had cooled, Boston life had begun to run in its usual seasonal channels, and the word inoculation had begun to fade out of the daily conversation. Before it disappeared, however, it had stamped two figures indelibly on Boston's memory — eight hundred and forty-four deaths and two hundred and eighty lives saved by inoculation. Without need of one more argument or the publication of one more pamphlet, these two figures had wrought a change in the public attitude, in spite of all the doubts and questions that still remained. Eight hundred and forty-four places at Boston's firesides were vacant. Two hundred and eighty men and women who had taken the risk were back behind their counters, at their desks, in their shops, or at home, and all were enjoying their usual health.

Zabdiel Boylston, so lately under heavy abuse and angry disfavor, had found through the early months of 1722 that his practice had not only been restored but had increased. His friends no longer felt obliged to defend him, and when it became known on the street that Sir Hans Sloane had invited Boylston to visit London as the guest of the Royal Society, he began to receive congratulations.

From February 24 to March 22, 1724, he advertised in the Boston *Gazette* that he would like to let his "good convenient Garden" — two and a quarter acres in extent, planted with fruit trees of various sorts, gooseberries, currants, a large asparagus bed, and sundry other plants and roots of value to a garden — and also sell at his shop, "saffron, Jollop root, good Cassia fistula, Juniper Berries, with other Druggs & Medicines at reasonable rates."

In the *Gazette* for July 29 to August 3, he inserted an advertisement which read, "These are to desire All Persons indebted unto Doctor Zabdiel Boylston to (send or come) and pay their Debts. And likewise to desire all Persons who have any demands on said Boylston to bring in their Accounts and receive their Money, he designing in a short time a voyage for London." The last item in this advertisement would suggest to his patients that he intended to return in due time. It read, "If any Persons have any Bear's Grease to sell, the said Boylston will give them 8/s per Gallon, for more or less." (Bear's grease was a needed item in a physician's supply of aids to health.)[1]

He sailed in December 1724, and remained in England for a year and a half, apparently his only period out of New England. It was a time of rich experience, especially for the opportunity it afforded him to confer with English physicians and other professional men at the Royal Society. His association with Sir Hans Sloane and Dr. James Jurin, Secretary of the Society, ripened into warm, personal friendships which continued long afterward. Boylston also satisfied his desire to study the new method "of cutting for the Stone" — his own particular specialty in surgery. He refused to inoculate as he was often urged to do, but he shared in the discussions and demonstrations at meetings of the Society and finally yielded to Sir Hans Sloane's importunate request that he write the story of his inoculations in Boston. He devoted the latter part of his time in London to doing so. The book was published in London in 1726 and reprinted in Boston both in that year and in 1730 when smallpox came again.

His election to the Royal Society came on May 26, 1726. He was proposed by Dr. J. B. Steigentahl. The Council approved, and on July 7, 1726, he signed the Obligation and was formally admitted as a Fellow of the Society. The record in the *Journal-Book* reads:

Zabdiel Boylston (March 9, 1679/80–March 1, 1766) Boston physician famed for his intelligent use of inoculation for smallpox in 1721–22 went to England in 1725 to study "the new method for cutting the Stone." Carrying a letter of introduction from Cotton Mather to Dr. James Jurin, Secretary of the Society, Boylston became Jurin's close friend and was occasionally guest at the Society's meeting. On May 26, 1726, Boylston was recommended by Dr. J. G. Steigentahl, for election to the Society. The Council approved, and on the same day Boylston was elected, signed the Obligation, and was formally admitted Fellow of the Society.[2]

The prime purpose of the Society, inherited from its predecessor, the "Invisible College," was "the accurate collection, classification, and interpretation of scientific data from all parts of the world." Candidates for admission promised "to promote the good of the Royal Society for improving natural knowledge, and to pursue the ends for which the same was founded." They promised also to attend meetings as far as was convenient, to pay weekly contributions of one shilling "toward the charges of Experiments, and other expenses of the Society, within four weeks after election, to appear in person before the Society, to pay an admission fee of forty shillings, and to be admitted by the President.[3]

Prior to Boylston's election, seven other New Englanders had been elected.

John Winthrop the Younger, 1661	John Leverett, 1713
William Penn, 1681	Elihu Yale, 1717
William Byrd, 1696	Paul Dudley, 1721
William Burnet, 1705	Cotton Mather, 1723
Thomas Nicolson, 1706	Thomas Robie, 1725[4]
Thomas Hay, 1707	Zabdiel Boylston, 1726
William Brattle, 1713 (declined)	
Walter Douglas, 1713/1714	

He was the twelfth American to be honored in the eighteenth century and the fifteenth since the founding of the Society in 1661. Boylston made only two contributions to the Royal Society's accounts of strange natural phenomena after his election. One concerning ambergris in whales was printed in the same year of his election, 1726, and reported in some detail the mystery of the bag in which the ambergris is found. He located it as "near the Genital Parts of the fish," but without any outlet or inlet to it and sometimes found quite empty. He ended his brief account with characteristic modesty. Whether or not "the ambergris be naturally or accidentally produced in that Fish, I leave to the Learned to determine." This spermaceti whale had been killed by Mr. Atkins of Boston, assisted by Mr. Greenleaf of Nantucket. Paul Dudley, member of the Royal Society, had also sent an account of this whale, included in the same volume of the *Philosophical Transactions*.

Zabdiel Boylston's second contribution concerned a large stone found in the stomach of a horse. A letter to Boylston about this stone is among the preserved correspondence of Sir Hans Sloane, President of the Society. "The stone," Sloane wrote, "was one of the largest I have seen. I have indeed several the smaller, unless one pretending to be a bezoar, from a horse, which is much bigger. I showed it to the Royal Society, who ordered me to give you their thanks."

The last sentence of this letter from Sloane reads, "I hope you will remember to give us notice here of what you find curious, which will be extremely grateful to your most obedient and most humble servant, Hans Sloane,"[5] Boylston's later observations on the rattlesnake and the failure to keep him alive all winter apparently did not get as far as a reply.

No more of his contributions were published by the Society, although the correspondence appears to have continued. As he stated in his *Historical Account*, "Writing is a Talent which of all Things, I never made any Pretentions to" but in the narrative of his Boston inoculations in 1721, written during the last days of his London

visit, he left a valuable record which tells much of his personal distinction as a physician, as well as reporting typical stages in the illness following inoculation. Aside from this account, a physician's
record of the outbreak of 1721 exists in mere scraps. Dr. Douglass
spoke of keeping a record of his many smallpox cases, but apparently
this account is not extant. His two discussions of inoculation came
ten years later, during the outbreak of 1730.

One priceless personal story of Zabdiel Boylston's year in London
has fortunately been preserved in print. It comes from Ward Nicholas Boylston, who in 1783 met Benjamin Franklin at Franklin's seat
just outside Paris. At that time Benjamin Franklin was seventy-
seven years old. His distinguished career was largely behind him,
and he had only seven more years to live. When he heard the name
Boylston called, he arose from his chair, and extending his hand,
said,

> "I shall always revere the name, Boylston. Sir, are you of the
> family of Zabdiel Boylston?"
>
> "Yes," answered Ward Nicholas. "He was my great-uncle."
>
> "Then sir, I must tell you," Franklin replied. "I owe every-
> thing I am to him. When Dr. Boylston was in London in
> 1726, I was there and reduced to the greatest distress, a youth
> without money, friends or counsel. I applied in my extreme dis-
> tress to him, who supplied me with twenty guineas, and relying
> on his judgment, I visited him as opportunities offered, and by
> his faithful counsels and encouragements I was saved from the
> abyss of destruction which awaited me, and my future fortune
> was based on his timely assistance.
>
> "Sir, I beg you will visit me as often as you find you have
> leisure while in Paris."[6]

Ward Nicholas did so, dined with Franklin several times, and
always received his marked attentions.

At the time of this youthful appeal, Franklin had been eighteen years old, had come to London for the first time with James Ralph, a Philadelphia companion, who had borrowed all Franklin's reserve cash and departed without paying the debt. What makes the story even more revealing of Boylston is that Franklin had been in Boston at the time of the inoculation quarrel and had written some of the cruel comment that his brother, James Franklin, had printed in the *New England Courant,* and probably Boylston had not forgotten that Franklin had done so. If Boylston had remembered that far-off chapter of indignity in 1726, it would have mattered not at all. He bore no grudges.

IX

Zabdiel Boylston's
An Historical Account, 1726

THE ACCOUNT that Boylston wrote, at the request of Sir Hans Sloane, of his own medical service in Boston during the 1721 outbreak of smallpox is in the form of a first-person story. Originally printed in London in 1726, it was reprinted in Boston in the same year and reissued in 1730, when smallpox came again. In his dedication to Caroline, Princess of Wales, Boylston called it "a faithful Narrative of my Practice in New England, at a Time when the Small Pox raged in that Country with the utmost Violence, and carry'd off great Numbers in a Week."

His book is exactly what he called it — a record of his two hundred and forty-seven cases of inoculation in 1721 with precise observation, very little detail, and emphasis on the success or failure of the operation in each case. The fact that it is the experience of one man, written at one time, many months after the events of that stormy year, gives it a unity, a detachment, and perspective that add to the value of the record. These much abbreviated, repetitious case histories also tell, perhaps unconsciously to the writer, more than they say, bringing alive on almost every page much of the atmosphere of this time of crisis in beleaguered Boston.

It begins on June 26 with the inoculation of his six-year-old son Thomas. This was Boylston's first inoculation and very probably one of his first experiences with a smallpox patient. Although in the 1702 outbreak, when he was twenty-two years old, he was a victim of the disease and almost lost his life, his medical career had not yet begun. Several years previously he had become an apprentice in the office of Dr. John Cutler, and several years later (1705) set up his own practice in Dock Square. Although forty-two years old in 1721, with some sixteen years of successful practice behind him, he confesses to "a very great fright" when his son's fever and that of little Jacky, son of his slave Jack, increased on the eighth day and Tommy's twitchings and startings in his sleep also increased. "I had nothing to have Recourse to but Patience, and therefore waited upon Nature for a Crisis (neither my Fears nor the Symptoms abating) until the 9th." He used means, whereupon "the Symptoms went off, a kind and favorable Small-Pox came out, of about an hundred a piece; after which their Circumstances became easy, our Trouble was over, and they were soon well."[1]

Over and over, the same favorable ending is repeated until it becomes almost a formula, but more regularly there is also some individual detail to make the patient something of a special person and to give a three-dimensional character to the brief story. For example, there is Joshua Cheever, an early patient, who came to Boylston on July 12, shortly after the frightening Dalhonde report. He was thirty-nine years old, "strong and lusty," and yet on the ninth day after inoculation, when the eruption had not appeared, Dr. Boylston concluded the inoculation had not been successful. The fire gong sounded, Joshua jumped out of bed, ran to the fire, climbed ladders, carried pails of water, removed the house furnishings, personal belongings, became overheated, and returned home full of pain and very ill. In the morning, Dr. Boylston found him "under the signs of a high fever, with a hard and quick Pulse," and feared he might have the confluent smallpox, the most dangerous sort. He was bled, purged, blistered, upon which "the Symptoms went off, the Small-Pox came out, of a kind, distinct Sort, his Pains and our Fears were soon over and in a short time he was well."[2] This is a quite typical entry, a setting for the case, a few details of the patient and the treatment, the favorable ending. When serious complications were present, and for the six patients who died, the story is told more fully.

Dr. William Douglass in his two pamphlets on inoculation made much of the proper preparation of the patient, avoidance of cold weather for the operation, and the strict necessity of quiet and no crowding in the sick room. Dr. Boylston knew of the desirability of such conditions, but he also knew how to face the reality of large families, lack of space, and parental pleading that could not be denied, as when he was called to the home of Edward Dorr, where he inoculated Father Edward and three of his children, but refused five more — three of them children, an Indian girl, and Dorr's servant man — until five days later. All these new patients were in the same room with the previously inoculated three, the Indian girl just behind the partition. The servant man is not specifically located.

By the time the first three were broken out for a day or two, the other five began their sickness. Here was a melancholy sight indeed. "I had often three or four, but never five in a Room together." Dr. Boylston's word, "the poor Children with their sickness, the Winter's Cold, prov'd froward, one crying, another coughing, one wanted Drink, one to get up, another to go to Bed, and so on; so that with opening of Doors, the gingling of the Warming-pan, Fire-shovel and Tongs, there was scarce a minute in all the 24 Hours that all was still and quiet." No wonder that Mr. Dorr, "his Pock inflam'd and his Fever too high, his great Concern for his Children, the continual Noise, and want of Sleep, made the poor Gentleman almost distracted . . ." obliged me "to bleed him twice, to apply Epispastics, use Anodines, &c. at the turning of the Pock. The Symptoms went off, the Indian girl was lost, but the other eight survived."[3]

Various comments show Boylston learning as he worked. Very early he discarded the Turkish method of covering the incision with half a nut shell. Instead, he used a cabbage leaf which he found to be better. He also changed the mere scratch on the arm to an incision through the "true skin" and then bound up the slight wound. Another comment concerns the difference he discovered between the natural and inoculated disease in various typical symptoms. He observed that the natural remained in the body longer than the inoculated before the eruption came. He raised the question why but had no answer. Again, how does the disease enter the body in the natural way of infection? Cotton Mather helped with this question later with his own inspired guess that the "animated particles" he saw with the "glass" were *animalculae,* alive and looking for their prey.

One of Dr. Douglass's criticisms of Boylston was that he did not screen his patients properly and reject those in feeble health. Had those he tried to dissuade taken his suggestion, perhaps at least four of the six who died might have escaped. Mrs. Dixwell, to whose case Boylston returned several times, was "a fat gentlewoman of a tender Constitution," who came to him frightened, having lived near those infected and having passed "for some days before a Door where lay a Corpse ready for the Grave." The weather also changed, she took cold, her condition became worse and in spite of "many Means used, she died on the 26th Day after Inoculation." John White, Esq., a weak, infirm man, "had insisted, in spite of Dr. Boylston's remonstrance, that he be inoculated. The smallpox came out on the ninth day, as usual, "the symptoms easy, except that he was splenetic and dull." Again on the twelfth and thirteenth, "it came forward again, tho slowly and of an indifferent Complexion." Now his "splenetic Darknesses" increased. He would take no nourishment . . . and refused to be spoken to or be comforted, "notwithstanding he had no Complaints either of Pain or Sickness, Heat or Oppression at his Breast. Thus he lay languishing, and withering away like a Plant without Moisture . . . until the 12th of Eruption and 21st from Inoculation, when he died."[4]

The typical cases are treated more briefly. "I inoculated the honourable Judge Quincy's Son, Mr. Edward Turil, Mr. Ebenezer Gee, each 18, Mr. Samuel Dunbar, 16, Mr. Samuel Freeman, 15, Mr. Benjamin Fitch, and Mr. James Varney, each 14, Mr. Edward

Wigglesworth, 32 (Mr. Hollis's Professor), Mr. William Welsteed, Fellow, 24, Mr. Benjamin Gibson, 21 years old. The Honourable Judge *Sewall's* Grandson, *Samuel Hirst,* 17, the Honourable *Jonathan Belcher's* Son *Andrew,* 15, Mr. James *Pitts,* 14 Years old. Meeting in this Practice, within three Days such a Number of our College Young Gentry (and with them two of their Overseers) I take the Liberty of mentioning them as such, and hope the Youths will manage well. Fifteen of these had the Small Pox at the usual Time, and of a kind, distinct Sort, few in Number, and their Symptoms gentle. Mr. *Wigglesworth,* had the Small Pox at the same time, and of a very distinct Sort, but not so kind; between the coming out and filling of the Pock, he suffer'd two or three Days, an Oppression of the Spirits, wandering Pains, and Sickness at Stomach, which all went off at the Ripening of the Pock, and he with the other Fifteen, soon recovered and did well."[5]

On this page, and also on several others, the names of the ministry, the college, the officialdom of Boston, suggest the support thinking men and women were giving Boylston during this time when newspaper columns were still soliciting and printing opposition. Francis Foxcroft, Samuel Danforth, Nehemiah Walter — ministers and influential men, all three — were helping to turn the tide of hostile criticism, but they were not doing it in newspaper columns. Yet, Zabdiel Boylston knew that he had their enthusiastic, favorable opinion behind him.

There are also many servant names in this list, both black and white — doubtless many unknown names. We know them by their symptoms and by the number of eruptions: "a generous sprinkling," a "handsome sprinkling," or "just a few." Very often the doctor counts them, "about a hundred," maybe "of a good, distinct color." He also reports those upon whom the operation had no effect. When Mr. Bent had no eruption on the ninth day, and it was assumed he must be inoculated a second time, a "Gentlewoman appeared and declared that she had seen him sick of the smallpox when he was a child." Few others remembered anything of it and his mother had been dead a long time. A servant girl of fifteen who broke out immediately after being inoculated, and only with great care was saved after the confluent type of smallpox had ended, confessed that she had gone into an infected house some time previously but had been afraid to tell it "for fear of Anger."

A group of men from Roxbury — Mr. Thomas Walter, Mr. Aspinwall, Mr. Dana — all lay in one room for the operation, and at the usual time they went through the whole process safely. On their return home their recommendation of the practice was such that forty more men inoculated at or near Roxbury were also saved, while of fourteen men who had the disease in the natural way at the same time, ten died.

So the story goes on and on through the two hundred and forty-seven cases. Twenty more pages give a table, a discussion of treatment, cautions, nursing care, food, medicine, and other details.

Perhaps Dr. Boylston's own confident assertion about inoculation after this experience is worth quoting. He wrote:

> Now if there be any one that can give a faithful Account or History of any other Method of Practice that has carried a Number, of all Ages, Sexes, Constitutions, and Colours, and in the worst Seasons of the Year, thro' the Small Pox; or, indeed, thro' any other acute Distemper with better Success, then I will alter my Opinion of this; and until then, I shall value and esteem this Method of Inoculating the Small-pox as the most beneficial and successful that ever was discover'd to, and practiced by Mankind in the World.[6]

X

War of Words

BOSTON'S WAR OF WORDS over inoculation, which had begun on June 26, 1721, with Zabdiel Boylston's first use of it, did not cease when fear of contagion had begun to be eased in early spring, 1722. Week by week during the preceding eight months, the columns of the *New England News Letter,* the Boston *Gazette,* and after August 7, the *New England Courant* had given space to this public quarrel. As it continued, now that life was beginning to be normal again, discussion became somewhat more discursive and less personal.

Very little of this voluminous expression of hasty opinion, especially in the earlier and again in the last stage, can be called controversy in the sense of serious debate. As long as near panic had the community in siege, almost everyone spoke too soon and too angrily. One-sided opinion found a newspaper column as soon as the types could be set. Frightened spokesmen could not wait even one day to express a vehement *no* to inoculation.

From beginning to end there were only two issues: Is inoculation safe for the patient, and does it insure immunity from future contagion? Neither question could be answered in a day; hence the comment wandered in byways, filling pages, differing from one source to the next only in vehemence of anger or surface details. There were as yet not enough facts; there could be no valid arguments, no tight reasoning, although both words were often used.

To look backward through these hundreds of pages, to find hints of growth toward a basis for sound conclusions is disappointing. Instead, most of it is a chaos of unsupported opinion with little knowledge behind it. What was needed at the outset was information, and this was at once supplied. The voice was Cotton Mather's. On June 22 he wrote in his diary:

> I prepare a little Treatise on the Small Pox, first remembering the Sentiments of Piety which it calls for, then exhibiting the best Medicines and Methods, which the world has yett had for the managing of it; and finally, adding the new Discovery, to prevent it in the way of Inoculation. It is possible that this Essay may save the Lives, and the Souls of many People. Shall I give it to the Booksellers? I am waiting for Direction.[1]

Of course he gave it and henceforth kept right on giving repetitions of the two articles published by the Royal Society. The titles differed, but the content was always the same. His pen was never idle. There is no anger in any of these treatises. He merely gives information, always staying close to the text of the Timonius and Pylarinus letters, adding his own unqualified assurance of their truth and accuracy. In his willingness to accept what he found in print without the shadow of a doubt, he was, of course, a man of his own day, as were most of his readers. But convincing information as to inoculation for a Boston audience at this date was a hard assignment — harder than Cotton Mather himself could quite realize.

Timonius and Pylarinus, after all, were not Bostonians. Timonius was a Turk, which is to say, he was a heathen, and whatever his medical advice, it was not for Christian Boston. Pylarinus was not much better. He had gathered all he knew from heathen, and as for inoculation itself, such instant revulsion as Boston residents would have felt in 1721 at the thought of inserting smallpox virus into the arms of their children is hard for a modern reader to understand. The hideousness, to say nothing of the danger, of smallpox was not a fact on the printed page for them. The unforgettable pictures were a part of nearly every family history for all but the youngest reading generation, creating a hostility of response from the very title of the pamphlet before them.

The *Little Treatise* of the diary entry was not printed under that title but appeared later, in greater part, in Chapter XX of *The Angel of Bethesda,* printed for the first time in 1972. The first of Mather's treatises that Bostonians read in print in 1721 was *Some Account of what is said of Inoculating or Translating the Smallpox,* "by the Learned Dr. Emanuel Timonius and Jacobus Pylarinus, To which are added a few Remarks and Quaeries thereon," published with Mather's permission, or more probably by his instigation, by Dr. Boylston. The Boylston remarks are easily separated from the Mather text, and in the storm of early protest against Boylston, these statements may have invited at least curiosity but did not redeem the pamphlet for most readers.

Mather's later *Account of the Method and Success of Inoculating the Small-Pox in Boston in New England* dedicated to Sir Hans Sloane and signed by Jeremiah Dummer, to whom Mather had given it for publication in London, is said to have been read with interest in England and to have had some influence at the time.[2] This pamphlet contains the Onesimus story and tells of meetings in Boston with other Africans who corroborated his statement of inoculation as a tribal custom. On October 30 Mather also printed *A Faithful Account of what has occurr'd under the late experiments of Small-Pox managed and governed in the way of Inoculation,* written when the fury of opposition was at its height. Mather says he wants "partly to put a stop to the unaccountable way of lying which fills the Town and County on this Occasion and partly for the Information & Satisfaction of our Friends in other Places."[3] The disease was at peak severity and a death from inoculation had made public interest very alert. The bomb thrown through Mather's window shortly after this pamphlet appeared added new strain.

Other combatants who deserve mention in this paper warfare include Benjamin Colman, pastor of the Brattle Street Church, who wrote *Some Observations on the New Method of Receiving the Small-Pox by Engrafting or Transplantation, containing also the Reasons which first Induc'd him to, and have since confirmed him in his favorable Opinion of it.*[4] Of all the many pamphlets written during these critical months, this is easily the best and the most successful. It appeared to convince many readers that inoculation was a reasonable practice.

Benjamin Colman's success would seem to have come from his frank layman's attitude. He made no pretense to medical knowledge and did not mind showing his ignorance. He tells simply what he saw as he went from house to house, visiting members of his flock. If he is scoffed at for telling this simple story, that is not important. "I do not think I go out of my way in this present Essay."[5] He describes the symptoms as he has observed them. "So gentle and perfect is Nature in this its own work without the assistance of medicine, and almost any need of nursing. Neither is there need of a Watcher by night, no more than of a Nurse by day. It moderates the first fever and seems totally to prevent the second."

One feels the modesty of this man who has come to a new idea with an open mind, not to accept or reject it, but to observe for himself. He had lived through these weeks of strain in Boston, apparently without taking sides. Firsthand evidence was his sole purpose, and the evidence seems to have persuaded him. "What an astonishing Mercy to us in this land this Discovery might prove," he exclaimed.

He keeps strictly to observed fact, in going from house to house, "whereby I (so far as I am) in favor of this Method, so much spoken against by so many."[6] He wins by having no other purpose than "to seek the truth and to be willing to learn it of the poorest Slave in the Town." His remark, "It may be scarce anyone has seen more than I," was a help in his criticism of himself and his brother ministers as probably spreading the contagion more than the inoculated, as had already been noted by critics. There was enough poison, he said, in one of these chambers to infect the whole town, and "why aren't the ministers carrying it with us?" Truly enough, and it was high time they realized it. His remark about the "animated atoms" revealed "in the glass" echoes Cotton Mather's statement. Presumably the two men had compared observations.

The religious scruples of some Bostonians as to inoculation were the subject of a pamphlet written by Willaim Cooper, associate pastor with Colman in the Brattle Street Church. It was entitled *A Letter to a Friend in the Country*. Cooper lists twelve of these objections, and then one by one answers them as simply as worried parishioners had asked them. The questions may amaze a modern reader, but they were very urgent to a devout worshipper in the pew at this time of crisis in Boston. Interest in Cooper's pamphlet lies mainly in his willingness to take these objections seriously, as though they were worth asking and worth a pastor's best care to put such worries out of the people's minds. Edmund Massey's sermon in London entitled "The Dangerous and Sinful Practice of Inoculation" was largely responsible for these questions. Its reprint in Boston had not created so much unrest as in English congregations, but enough to make such a rebuttal as Cooper's pamphlet worth doing. The simple kindness of his answers quieted the fears Massey's sermon had raised in Boston and may have done the same in London, where this pamphlet was also reprinted immediately.[7]

The contrast between the sensationalism Massey's fears had raised and the simplicity of Cooper's answers emphasizes two ways of thinking about the ways of God with man that presaged sermon battles yet to come. Massey interpreted his Bible literally. His protagonist, Job, had been smitten with boils from the crown of his head to the soles of his feet. The devil had infused such a poison into his body that his blood had been raised to a ferment that caused "a confluence of inflamatory Pustules," just as inoculation does. Certainly, and why not? Timonius and Job lived in the same country,

and this "venemous infusion" might, in fact, have been the same —
the very same — as inoculation. God took away the boils when
Job's faith met the test. Diseases are God's business, not man's.
Men are trying to take God's power away from him. Dire sin this
is. Let atheists inoculate. Let God's people bless God for his afflictions upon us. Cooper was content to say very simply, "Let us use
the light God has given us and thank him for it." William Cooper
was a sensible man and laid each of the twelve objections to rest
quietly without torturing a Biblical analogy in the process.

After August 1721, the tone of the Boston pamphlet discussion of
inoculation changed in partial response to that of the *New England
Courant,* Boston's third newspaper, whose first issue appeared on
August 7. James Franklin, founder of this new sheet, had learned
while he was in London studying the printer's trade that wit and
satire helped the subscription returns, and he decided to try this resource for his newspaper. In his second issue, August 14, he invited
his readers to favor him with "some short Pieces, Serious, Sarcastic,
Ludicrous, or other ways amusing, or sometimes profusely *DULL,*
to accommodate some of his Acquaintance." There was one condition. He would print nothing "reflecting on the Clergy of whatever
Denomination." This condition deceived no one, not even Cotton
Mather, whom Franklin hated without qualification.

The short pieces came, both sarcastic and ludicrous, but so em-
barrassingly barren of wit as not to deserve the label of even the
palest sort of amusement. It accomplished nothing except to increase
antiministerial sentiment with a blunt literalness that became a
feeble bore. The contributors, mostly anonymous, lacked the
subtlety and the dexterity to handle such materials skillfully enough
to raise a laugh, and they quickly fell back on name-calling or ex-
aggerations of the ministerial jeremiad which Boston had heard in
election sermons for a generation. Also, the increased number of
deaths, as the smallpox infection reached its peak in September,
October, and early November, made this pseudocomic accent out of

place. In addition, the ministerial response unfortunately began to echo the ironic new strain and attempted to respond bluntly and literally.

One pamphlet which may well represent this unwise attempt to regain the ministerial leadership of earlier times in the governance of New England affairs was the anonymous pamphlet entitled *A Vindication of Some Ministers of Boston from the Abuses and Scandals, lately cast upon them in Diverse Printed Papers.*[8] The question, who wrote this vindication?, interested both sides in the inoculation quarrel more than the text of the piece itself. Benjamin Colman denied that he had any part in it, and he may well be believed, for neither the idea nor the tone has any resemblance to the spirit of any of his published pieces. Other ministers were also quickly absolved as all eyes continued to look in Cotton Mather's direction. In print his phrase for James Franklin had been "the wicked Printer," and for those who wrote for the *Courant,* "The Hell-Fire Club," so that the ascription of authorship to Mather seemed fair enough. Most of all, the style of the piece gave cause for the ascription. The opening reads:

> Boston may boast of almost an unparallel'd happiness in their ministers. Some of us have travell'd to other and diverse parts of the World and we sincerely profess, we never saw the Place that excelled Boston in this respect. God has indulged to this People, a very Candid, Learned, and Religious set of Men. Some of them have Great Names in distant Lands.
>
> And we thought our Neighbors were all sensible of the invaluable *Blessings* of God to us in this Regard, But to our Astonishment we see some in this Place so astonishingly Profane, as to libel, and lampoon the Holy Servants.[9]

Whoever wrote the *Vindication* did not see Cotton Mather's diary entry, written January 25–26, 1721/1722, which reads, "Something must be done towards the suppressing and Rebuking of those wicked Pamphlets that are continually published among us to lessen and blacken the Ministers and poison the People. Several Things of an exquisite Contrivance and Composure, are done for this Purpose. Tho my poor Hand is the doer of them, they must pass thro other Hands, that I may not pass for the Author of them."[10]

In this entry and various others, of course, Mather may be speaking of some piece other than the *Vindication,* but retributory action toward printed criticism was an admitted motive in something he wrote. An entry for January 16, six days earlier, reads, "The Villainous Abuses offered and multiplied unto the Ministers of this Place, require something to be done for their Vindication. I provide Materials." What happened, of course, was that the *Vindication* was answered, ridiculed, lampooned, as the anonymous author had invited it to be. It was probably talked over in the tobacco cellar of John Williams, nicknamed Mundungus, who had already evoked at least a few laughs by his publications, which were cast in syllogistic form — as he thought — with misspellings and always with a grain of common sense in them somewhere, but pitiful enough even so. A voice from his level belonged in this public quarrel, but it need not have borne the taint of unseemly language brought from the tobacco cellar.

The speakers in the finale of this long controversy were assembled by Isaac Greenwood, a young intellectual of Harvard, later to be Hollis Professor of Mathematics and Natural Philosophy. He called it *A Friendly Debate* between Academicus (Greenwood), Sawny (Dr. William Douglass), and Mundungus (John Williams of the tobacco cellar). Clever, within limits, at times mildly amusing, this piece deflates the importance of the inoculation discussion, ridicules Douglass unforgettably, but perhaps eased the strain of the long smallpox anxiety by the change of temper it supplied and also invoked. It is no more than an abusive skit in which Mundungus, the wag, comes off as a winner in the adroit handling by Isaac Greenwood. Of all the pieces written in this late, not so serious chapter of the controversy, this is the only one that meets to any degree James Franklin's plea for enlivening wit and satire.

In long sequel, this controversy had made scant progress toward clarifying the main issues, but it had introduced a new point of view in medical practice. It had put new power in men's hands in the control of disease and emphasized new responsibilities in community leadership.

The authority of ministerial leadership in secular affairs had been dealt a blow from which complete recovery could hardly be expected. The importance of ministers in the community would henceforth be in their own hands as individual citizens. It would not be pulpit power they would wield, such as previously had been recognized as authoritative.

As to victory for the physicians, strangely enough it would be expressed for a long future by Dr. William Douglass, leader of the opposition to inoculation during the crucial year, 1721. He had ventured no final statements in the year; he had abused Zabdiel Boylston, who began the practice in New England, well past forgiveness. As to inoculation itself, he said only time would tell. After nine years, he wrote two pamphlets giving a considerably changed verdict. The two pamphlets offered the clearest, soundest exposition of the new practice of any that appear in this long controversy, putting his modified verdict on scientific grounds so far as experiment had gone by 1730. Ultimate goals were not yet reached; he would not live to know how they were reached; he was speaking for 1730.

His two treatises are entitled *Dr. Douglass's Practical Essay Concerning the Small Pox,* Boston, 1730, and *A Dissertation Concerning Inoculation of the Smallpox,* London, 1730. A sample quotation from the *Dissertation* states his verdict, which would hold for a long time.

We find by some years' experience, that the Small Pox abstractly considered, received by Inoculation, is not so fatal, and the Symptoms frequently more mild, than in the accidental Contagion; yet it is not of that certain Safety, to exempt it from being precarious, and therefore requires Discretion in applying it to proper Subjects, and Judgment in managing the Distemper so received.[11]

During the 1730 outbreak in Boston, Douglass had used inoculation in his own practice, when his patients so desired.

XI

Two Generations
of Doubtful Practice

BOSTON'S RESPITE from smallpox after 1721, although rather brief, had brought nine years of peace and apparent prosperity, the turmoil and clamor long past, the controversy over, inoculation all but forgotten. The town's population had increased to fourteen thousand. The new residents knew nothing about the restraints of quarantine, the tolling of funeral bells all day long, red flags at infected houses up and down every street. Then on October 27, 1729, a brief item appeared in the *New England Journal* that the ministers of the town would observe a day of prayer and fasting on account of the imminent danger of smallpox. This time a ship from Ireland was suspected of bringing the disease. The announcement seemed unbelievable. The 1721 terror could not come again, but everybody watched.

For several weeks the *New England Journal* made no further mention of danger. Whisperings grew louder, and when another brief notice appeared stating that the courts would be moved because smallpox was in town, a general alarm followed. There were four thousand cases and five hundred deaths. Increased acceptance of inoculation, particularly by parents of young children, made a difference as did the fact that many adults had gained immunity in 1721. The honor shown to Dr. Boylston in London also had helped to quiet the earlier prejudice and to modify the public attitude toward inoculation. Boylston's book was reprinted in Boston and widely read. In a little more than a year, the outbreak was over though it had been unusually severe.

But that was not the last time. Other outbreaks, limited in scope and widely scattered, continued to come in places not previously affected. At Wallingford, Connecticut, in 1732, there were fifty cases and fourteen deaths; on Martha's Vineyard in 1737, forty-three cases and twelve deaths; in Newport, Rhode Island, in 1739, sixty-seven cases and seventeen deaths. The per cent of fatalities was high in each case, and though in New York, Charlestown, and Philadelphia many cases were reported, the disease did not become endemic as it had in even smaller centers in England.

Boston would have three more outbreaks, each approaching major proportions: in 1751–1752, 1764, and 1775–1776. More residents would flee the city each time, and of those who remained more were inoculated. Consequently each time the ratio of deaths was slightly lower, but the danger of death from inoculation still deterred many adults from taking the risk.

During the half century until 1750 various new laws, mainly concerned with stricter quarantine, were passed. The penalty for failure to put out a red flag at an infected house was increased. Magistrates were given power to remove patients suffering from any contagious disease to a quarantine hospital. The spread of contagion from inoculation was again the subject of discussion. Doctors warned in vain, for as soon as a patient's mild illness had ended, he "began to do all things at all times" scattering infection as he went.

The answer for Boston and other towns, both small and large, began to be the inoculation hospital and a more forcible insistence on a stated recovery period before release. The Suttons, father and son, in England, insisted on a thirty-day recovery period, announced an easier method for the operation, and raised their already high prices, thereby limiting prevention even more severely to all but the more leisured and sufficiently affluent. Boston took note of all this and began to imitate the Suttons.

The inoculation hospitals of Dr. Aspinwall in Brookline (he built three of them) survived until Dr. Jenner's discovery of cowpox vaccination which ended smallpox inoculation overnight. All three of these hospitals were excellently managed and had not only won for Dr. Aspinwall a wide respect as a notable physician, but also had helped to put inoculation on a stable, professional basis. Unfortunately this was not true of all such institutions at the time.

With the Massachusetts temper of the early 1770s, the Tea Party, and the many small uproars over liberty poles, it was assured from the moment an inoculation hospital was proposed in any town meeting in the whole area that some degree of violence would be active until the day the obnoxious structure was torn down or set on fire by night. Violence in one place parallels that in another, wherever a town record tells the story. Two examples are the reactions to the establishment of the Marblehead inoculation hospital built on Cat Island and the Essex Hospital in Salem, built on Great Pasture in the same year.

In both cases, political issues underlay the medical. The Marblehead promoters were four powerful Whig leaders: Elbridge Gerry, John and Jonathan Glover, and Azor Orne. Dr. Hall Jackson, who had been prominent in Boston's inoculation program during the outbreak of 1764, was hired as the inoculator. At almost the same time the Salem town meeting voted the construction of their hospital. Previously their selectmen had been making daily inspections and sending all persons with suspicious symptoms to the contagious hospital on Spectacle Island. Timothy Pickering, a young Whig leader in Salem with strong political ambitions, was a member of the Board of Overseers of the hospital and had a leading part in the town meeting vote to build it. He had voted for James Latham as inoculator, but was already suspicious of him. Latham was a complete stranger to Massachusetts who had come from New York Colony, represented himself as a business associate of the British Suttons (father and son), using the secret method they had sold to him but improving it by safer and more comfortable drugs. The Suttons were known to be lavish users of calomel, not a new drug at this time in American smallpox therapy, but known to cause patients considerable suffering. Hence, no doubt, Latham's announcement of different drugs.

Latham had no sooner begun to treat his first class of patients than an article appeared in the *Essex Gazette,* signed Marblehead and opposing the Sutton method, insisting it was in truth an American method not discovered by Sutton or even taken to England by him. The honor belonged to Dr. Hall Jackson, inoculator in Marblehead hospital.

"Americans," the Marblehead author implores, "resent such conduct. Show no countenance to a man who makes a mystery of that which you already know." The next issue of the *Essex Gazette* carried an article by Dr. Nathaniel Whitaker, minister of Salem's third church, supporting the Marblehead criticism of Sutton and going further. His system was a fraud, and he himself a blacksmith, not a physician at all. "No, a horse doctor. A British institution. No! The method is American." Whether the political flavor of this quarrel pleased *Essex Gazette* readers or not, political it had become.

Pickering's criticism of Latham increased, but he waited too long and lost his chance to act on it. The Salem hospital was completed in early December. The first class was enrolled on December first. There were one hundred and thirty-two patients. Much complaint was made of their suffering through the treatment. There was one death and one case of serious illness without hope of recovery. Meanwhile, newspaper articles were printed in New York favoring Latham, and these articles were reprinted by the New England press. A week after the second class had entered, Latham raised his prices. The overseers objected. Latham answered by agreeing to inoculate forty poor patients at half price and to hire an assistant at his own expense. Instead of suffering only a slight illness, his patients became very ill and a child died.

A patient who had been in class one had kept some of the pills. They were examined and found to be calomel. At this point, Pickering printed an article revealing what had been discovered. He withheld his name, signing himself "A Lover of Truth." Latham replied by challenging him to a duel. Pickering had the wit not to accept the challenge. After this, to hasten the end, smallpox broke out in the hospital. The town acted, ordering the institution closed permanently.[1] By this sad travesty on community protection, the cause of what at this date was the best-known way to save human beings from smallpox contagion was set back no less than twenty years.

The inoculation hospital on Cat Island had an equally sad ending with even more sensationalism along the way. Sturdy opposition dated from the day the town had voted to build it. A meeting to reconsider this vote was dissolved without a discussion, and the hospital was built, surrounded by fences and trenches to further safeguard against intrusion or escape. Deliveries were made to a special gate not used by patients; there were two hospital boats. There were a hundred and three patients in the first class, and opening day was a gala day in Marblehead.

The gala spirit was short-lived. Some patients left too early and were met by a mob at the water's edge. One of the hospital boats was burned. After the third class had been inoculated, smallpox broke out in the hospital. The town ordered the institution closed until the townspeople saw fit to reopen it. Four men who stole the clothing that was put out to air were caught and put in the Salem jail. A procession of one thousand marched to Salem and got them out. The four men were tarred and feathered and drawn to Marblehead in a cart to be exhibited.

John Glover, warned that his house would be attacked, put a loaded cannon in his hallway, opened the front door, and with the cannon turned on the throng, appeared with a lighted torch in his hand. Missiles were thrown at the closed hospital building, windows were broken, and much damage done. A tub of tar was brought in.

The hospital, equipped with seventy beds, was completely destroyed by fire.[2] Immediately the patriot cause, led by the four Whigs: Elbridge Gerry, John and Jonathan Glover, and Azor Orne — the proprietors of the Hospital Board — made front page news for Marblehead during the mid-seventies.

XII

Edward Jenner's *Inquiry*, 1798

EDWARD JENNER CAME late into the smallpox story, but he came at a time when a new chance was urgently waiting. By 1748, the year of his birth, inoculation had been saving thousands of lives for twenty-seven years. With many physicians in England, many parts of Europe, as well as in America, it had become almost a standard medical practice, willingly accepted by a growing number.

But it was still not good enough. Better preparation, as well as wiser care during the mild illness that followed, had decreased the number of deaths considerably, but one death in a hundred was still too many, and often there were more. Also, it could no longer be denied that wherever inoculation was used and no matter how carefully, smallpox contagion always spread. Neither strict quarantine nor inoculation hospitals could avail. Contagion defeated all measures taken to restrict it. Most serious of all, the increasingly elaborate preparation, with fees to match, and the longer recovery period that was required, had increased the cost until only a few could afford inoculation in either price or time. The poor and ignorant of the world were excluded. Furthermore, another change that was imperative was the restriction of the operation to a special physician, classified as an inoculator. Any physician was an inoculator when the need arose.

What was needed was the discovery of a safer medium and one plentiful enough to take care of all. Only when these two requirements were met, could inoculation be a universal privilege.

In modern times these requirements would be met through years of seclusion in a laboratory, financed by public grants. Edward Jenner's life was quite otherwise. He was a country doctor living a villager's life, amid the quiet fields and vales of Gloucestershire, a man without worldly ambition, to whom nature and nature's creatures were both setting and society. He was a man of simple tastes who served the country people for miles around, delighting them with his songs, his flute music, his impromptu verses, and also answering their questions on matters far afield, for he was a man of wide interests and rich stores of information, although not at all a man of books.

He entered the medical profession by the country door, when as a young boy he became apprenticed to a certain Mr. Ludlow, a surgeon of Sodbury. He might have chosen Oxford as his brother Stephen had done, but Gloucestershire was his first love, as it would continue to be throughout his life. He spent the next seven years in close daily association with a man who knew his country people, their diseases, their way of life, and expected from his young learner something akin to partnership within the limits of country practice. When amputation was required, the apprentice held the patient down, assisted with the dressings, took care of the instruments, and when the day's work was done, he roamed the fields, collected fossils, studied birds. Some day he would find out something no one else knew yet about the strange ways of the cuckoo, that would thereafter earn him his membership in the Royal Society. Jenner's eyes saw everything, his fingers grew nimble and obedient, and when the seven years were accomplished, he had learned what country patients and Mr. Ludlow could teach him. He had also learned that there was more to know about medicine.

In a current issue of a London newspaper, he saw the announcement of Dr. William Hunter's School of Anatomy, said to be the best-equipped institution of its kind in the world at that time and promising a full course of training in anatomy and physiology, as well as midwifery. What seemed especially to catch his imagination was a word about the school of anatomy where students could see everything that was going on, and with their own hands dissect as many bodies, make for themselves as many preparations, and perform as many operations of surgery as they please. When he learned that William Hunter's younger brother John, now surgeon at St. Joseph's Hospital, would take him as a student assistant for two years for a hundred pounds a year, he eagerly accepted.

In company with Stephen, his elder brother, Jenner set out for London by horseback and coach, a three days' journey, and found his way to Windmill Street, where the Hunter institution stood. He would live in John Hunter's house as his only student learner, walk the wards of St. Joseph's Hospital every morning with his teacher, watch him at work in the dissecting laboratory in the afternoons, and presently have some free time there himself. Apparently headed for a surgeon's career under a brilliant teacher, he would not know until years afterward that he was headed elsewhere.

One day while an apprentice with Mr. Ludlow, he had been impressed with the remark of an ungrown country girl, a milkmaid, who had come asking help for her hands which were broken out with pustular sores. "It can't be smallpox," she exclaimed, "for I've had the cow-pox and everybody knows you can't have the smallpox after that." Her remark passed out of Jenner's mind at the moment, and he did not know until long afterward that he had not forgotten it. Shortly before his death he remembered the occasion when he knew it had determined his life.

John Hunter had been an army surgeon before accepting the responsibility of St. Joseph's Hospital, with irregular training behind him, but already an enviable record of surgical success. He challenged almost everything his student learner had been taught by his country master, repeating over and over, "Experiment is the way to learn. Be sure of your facts, and never mind the opposition. Observation, patience, accuracy are the path to knowledge." Jenner also learned in the wards, day after day, as he watched and listened, that just curing the patient was not the only goal, but discovering new medical knowledge on his own initiative was as important. Take nothing for granted, Hunter kept on saying. If the cure doesn't come, don't blame the patient or the medicine; you didn't look accurately enough. Gradually, Jenner began to realize that experiment was replacing the long tradition in which he had been trained. Tradition meant less to men like Hunter, and the way of experiment was an open door. He was learning the greatest lesson of his life.

After two years he received his certificate testifying to "great diligence," and now on to physics, *materia medica,* and chemistry. During his second year he was asked to classify and arrange an exhibit of geology collected by Joseph Banks on a three-year voyage of exploration with Captain Cook in the *Endeavour.* Another three-year voyage was in prospect and Jenner was invited to go along as the associate of Joseph Banks. He refused at once. That was not his world. He also refused the offer of one General Smith, an army officer, en route to India for a period of residence. A chance to see the world and to live a leisured life of social pleasure. No, he was returning to Gloucestershire. John Hunter was disappointed that Jenner did not choose a surgeon's life in London, but he was too wise a man to try persuasion.

The companionship between master and pupil had become a warm friendship, which would continue for twenty years longer, as long as Hunter would live. His main interest was in comparative anatomy, and it was making his London house into a museum of sorts already. There was a stuffed camel in the hallway, a whale somewhere else, live leopards, and many smaller animals in cages with the number increasing daily. When he returned to Gloucestershire, Jenner sent his master many hedgehogs, while keeping a record of temperatures for more hedgehogs himself through the winter and supplying Hunter with many details of their hibernation, which was one of the research projects of the hour. A rare friendship enriched these two lives and gave the younger one the best possible introduction to creativity in his profession.

Back in Gloucestershire in a leisurely period (for Jenner was incapable of hurry), he built up a modest country practice, traveling on horseback to scattered patients, often too far for return overnight. In between there was plenty of time for the birds, for discovery of the murderous way of the day-old fledgling cuckoo, born in the hedge-sparrow's nest, and immediately pushing the just hatched sparrows out on the ground, so that he might claim all the tiny mother's attention for himself. He wrote a paper about his discovery, sent it to Hunter for criticism, and then postponed rewriting it for several more years.

Meanwhile, for a considerable period, Jenner engaged himself with pleasures of the countryside. One of these was the constructing of a small balloon, inflating it with gas, and then seeing it float successfully for some ten miles to the delight of a large company of country neighbors. To make this a better story, it ended with his marriage to Katharine Kingscote, whose hand had held the cord of the balloon until it was released. Also in this period he organized a medical society for young physicians of the neighborhood. The name Convivio-Medical Society suggests its social pleasures along with the intellectual. His interest in the standardization of certain popular drugs led him to make his own brand of tartar emetic, which promised success, but the fact that he did not manufacture it in sufficiently large enough quantities or patent it for sale meant that it was soon forgotten.

An outbreak of smallpox in the late 1770s brought the milkmaid's remark into sharp focus once more, and until he had proved this folk tradition to be scientific truth, it was a leading motivation in his thought and action. It was during this outbreak, when many were seeking inoculation for protection, that he found among them those upon whom the operation had no effect. One answer might be, he reflected, that they had had cowpox, but if so, it had not been remembered in this dairy country and was too incidental to have been recorded anywhere.

He began to talk with his neighbors. Neither the younger generation nor their parents had ever heard of the tradition. The grand-
parents knew of it, but no one had ever made the test. All that they
reported was that sometimes it seemed to work and sometimes it
didn't. There was no faith to be put in it. Once Jenner wandered
into a blacksmith shop where the owner was treating a horse with
heels affected with the disease known locally as the *grease.* Later,
when this same man milked the cow, the cow developed cowpox and
so did the milker. Inoculated with smallpox virus in the usual manner, the patient resisted the infection. Was this disease of the horse's
heels a kind of smallpox? Jenner found other cases similar to this
one, and for a time he was inclined to think he had hit upon a valuable clue, but nothing definitive came of it.

He began to study the cow and soon discovered that she had more
than one pustular disease. All of these were called cowpox, but they
were by no means the same. His study of cowpox proper was de-
layed over and over, for the disease was not seasonal, could never be
predicted, and at one time was absent from the entire neighborhood
for a two-year span. When cases were again available for study,
Jenner made a further discovery; namely, that the virus taken from
the same cow might at one time have the virtue of resisting the
smallpox inoculation and at another time would not have it. The
conclusion from this discovery was that like the smallpox virus, that
of cowpox changed at some point, thereby losing its protective
quality. To distinguish the effective from the impotent called for
more observation, experiment, and study.

When he had satisfied himself that he had recognized the difference, Jenner took a drawing master with him one day and had an
illustration made on a white skin and a dark skin example of a true
cowpox pustule. These examples proved helpful when later published in his book. Many months went by as these experiments and
studies continued. The queries asked over and over at the dairies, the
long journeys first to one and then to the other, the hours spent in

the cow barns, all amused some of Jenner's friends and bored others, but he persisted, until, as John Hunter would have said, he had all his facts straight, and the time for the determining tests had at last come.

But there would be more discouragements. His fellow physicians did not share his confidence that immunization would surely follow from inoculation with the cowpox virus. From the evidence he had collected, certainty was still lacking. Even John Hunter, to whom Jenner's project was interesting for Jenner's sake only, was unimpressed. But Edward Jenner was a resolute man, and though when the outbreak of 1792 had ended, and there was no cowpox reported anywhere in the neighborhood, he was understandably deeply depressed, he was by no means defeated. He decided to propagate the disease from one human being to another, after the first patient had been inoculated from the cow. He inoculated a boy named Phipps from a pustule on the arm of a girl who had been infected by one of her master's cows. To his surprise both pustules closely resembled those of cowpox in some of their stages. Subsequent inoculations of the boy with smallpox virus produced no effect whatever, to Jenner's great encouragement.

At this particular stage of strain, hope, or more discouragement, no cow would oblige, and it was the spring of 1796 when the new turn of experiments could continue. At that time, from a pustule on the teat of a cow, Jenner inoculated five-year-old William Summers, who developed a typical case of cowpox. This served as a source of inoculation for Hannah Excell, seven years old, and Edward Jenner's eleven-month-old son Robert was inoculated from the pustule on Hannah's arms. This was a test Jenner had waited to perform since the birth of the child. The series of human inoculations continued, and in every case the smallpox test proved ineffectual. No sign of smallpox appeared on any child's body.

Taking advice before going further, Jenner submitted his results to a committee of physicians, who advised sending the paper to the

Royal Society of which Jenner was now a member. This body re-
jected his paper as "too revolutionary." A blow indeed, but to the
mind of the committee of physicians further delay was nothing
short of criminal. Accordingly, with their support and his own firm
conviction that this last test was valid, he published his paper under
the title *An Inquiry into Cause and Effects of the* Variolae Vaccinae.
It sold for seven shillings and sixpence.

Nothing about it suggests that it is a book containing a great
secret — sixty-four pages with wide margins, more space than it
needs, often more words than it needs, and not always clear to the
unscientific reader. Like Cotton Mather's *Angel of Bethesda,* it begins by making the disease of man a consequence of his sin. By
1796 many readers were still under the thralldom of that sad idea.
But Jenner is no preacher, and he immediately asserts without qualification that the mild disease of cowpox protects the person who has
suffered it forever afterward from infection of the smallpox. His
positive and unqualified statement is followed by a list of cases in
which this protection has lasted for twenty-seven, forty-three, thirty-
eight, two years, and one year, without exception.

Another list follows of local children inoculated first from a pustule on the arm of Sarah Nelmes, and from her to James Phipps — a
first story that would be repeated times without number. Smallpox
inoculation being familiar to all readers at this time, there was no
need for explanation at this point, only for the number of advantages
cowpox inoculation possesses over the familiar operation. It causes
no contagion, produces no deformity in the skin, has never been
known to be fatal. In his investigation thus far, Jenner asserts
plainly:

> I have proceded in an inquiry founded on experiment and I
> shall continue to prosecute this inquiry, encouraged by the
> pleasing hope of its becoming essentially beneficial to man-
> kind.[1]

To say it in less exciting phrase would be a problem for a master in the use of English. As a matter of fact, the first readers were not excited.

Jenner knew that demonstrations would now be in order and before the book had come from the press, he repaired to London to await the throng who would most certainly come. The next sentence is hard to write for nobody came. Precisely what his own anticipation had been one cannot surmise, but surely in addition to his own satisfaction that he had proved his point, he must have known that great things would come of it, that eventually the world would be without smallpox and without danger to anyone in the medium of protection used. But there was no reaction whatever as three months passed. It is true he was an unknown country doctor. William and John Hunter had died. He had few friends in London, and he had done nothing whatever to advertise his coming. The unpretentious little book of sixty-four pages had been published and presumably read by a few.

He had brought with him a small quill with matter from the arm of Hannah Excell. He left this with Dr. Cline, a friend, surgeon at St. Thomas's Hospital. Dr. Cline at the time had a boy patient with an inflamed hip joint, and thinking that the matter in the quill would give the boy the counterirritant his case required, he inserted the virus and got the results he wanted. Dr. Lister, a physician in the smallpox hospital, watched the case and was convinced it was not possible to give the boy smallpox. Dr. Cline wrote a letter to Jenner telling him of this confidence. After Jenner's death, this letter was found in his journal and fastened to it was a note written by Jenner telling of the confidence given him by Cline's letter, namely, from the fact that the matter had not lost its virtue after having been sealed up in the quill for three months. Dr. Lister immediately published what had happened. The London press spread it far and wide at once, sharply dividing the medical world, and causing an unseemly quarrel with Jenner expressly at the center. One of the first bombs came from the imperial physician to the Emperor of Austria, Dr. Ingenhouse, who, knowing nothing about cowpox (for it did not occur in Austria), found a farmer in Wiltshire who testified that he had had smallpox thirty years after having cowpox. Other opposers found other cases. There was nothing gained by trying to answer them, and besides, Jenner's supporters gave him even more trouble. Dr. Pearson, seeing the possibilities of fame and fortune, immediately issued a pamphlet of commendations he had solicited, and immediately afterward, an offer to supply physicians with the cowpox matter. Very quickly the impression was afloat that Pearson was the discoverer of cowpox inoculation.

Another supporter, Dr. Woodville, physician in charge of the smallpox hospital at Paddington, gave a demonstration in Cray's Inn, London, got his lancets mixed and soon had a smallpox outbreak on hand. There was no malice in Dr. Woodville and no excess of personal ambition. He was either excited or careless, but he learned, and in time helped the cause. As for Dr. Jenner, he realized at once that a new edition of his book was called for and that his presence in London was important.

The new version was more emphatic as to the possibility of spurious cowpox matter and also of the need to take it at the proper time — before its protective character had changed. Experience was the teacher in both cautions. Dr. Pearson was one who had not yet learned, when he supplied matter for fourteen patients at the Edgeworth Estate during the summer of 1799. All became gravely ill of smallpox and there was one death. Still later Pearson organized a vaccine board and even offered Jenner a post on it as extra-corresponding member. Needless to say, this offer was declined with the proper dignity.

The later story of Jenner is the world's story.[2] The old inoculation was gone overnight. The cry for the new vaccine came from all corners of the world and became a moving story for each country. Jenner himself tried to answer India's importunate call by sending eighteen children to be inoculated in turn during the voyage so that the vaccine might be kept fresh through the long journey. But Vienna had a better way — supply India by using Constantinople as a station for inoculation on the way. By sailing ships on the sea, by horses and camels on dry land, the quills full of the vaccine went everywhere.

Jenner's life became the life of a letter-writer — answering hundreds of inquiries, criticisms, protests, cautions without end — keeping him out of the fields for months of every year. At the time of the migration of birds, however, he usually managed to be back in Gloucestershire for a too brief time, as he missed the country life bitterly. For all the days he had left, his would be a life without leisure, without peace, with appearances before royalty, always throngs of people, a gold medal now and then, an honorary degree from Oxford, friends without number. But there was always jealousy, as rival claimants tried to take his discovery away from him. Somehow Jenner maintained serenity through it all.

XIII

Benjamin Waterhouse's Campaign in Boston

DR. BENJAMIN WATERHOUSE is important in Boston's smallpox story as the self-appointed herald of Jennerian vaccination at a time and to a public not yet ready to accept it. Fortunately he had advantages for this difficult role. He had a better medical education than most American physicians of his generation. He was forty-five years old and for sixteen years had been professor of the Theory and Practice of Physic in Harvard College. His appointment to this post had come with the establishment of a department of medicine in the college. During the past sixteen years he had more than once declared himself a firm advocate of the new method of experimental investigation in medicine, and although some of the younger physicians were alert and listening, many of their older colleagues were still safely conservative and following traditional opinion and practice.

In 1799 Waterhouse received from Dr. John Coakley Lettsom, an English physician, a copy of Edward Jenner's *Inquiry,* published the preceding year. Dr. Lettsom was also in the van of experimental medical thinkers. Shortly Waterhouse also received Dr. Pearson's endorsement of Jenner's discovery and the account of Dr. Woodville's experiments with cowpox inoculation. Having read Jenner's book and the two enthusiastic reports of the new practice, Dr. Waterhouse wrote and printed on the front page of Boston's *The Columbian Centinel* a brief article entitled "Something Curious in the Medical Line." His word *curious* put him back more than a hundred years to the time when the Royal Society had sent appeals to every corner of the earth requesting eyewitness accounts of the *curious* behaviors of nature, something unusual, unexpected, in fact, *curious*.

His article, though it would have met this requirement, attracted very slight interest. It announced cowpox as a pustular disease of cows, unknown in America, but familiar in certain parts of England, particularly in Gloucestershire. Milkers of infected cows contracted the disease, which produced a slight illness and caused an eruption on their hands, similar to that on the teats of the cows. After a few days the eruption disappeared and the illness was forgotten, but it had now been discovered and proved by Dr. Jenner that those who had suffered this mild disease were forever afterward protected from smallpox infection. No deaths had ever occurred from the cowpox.

The limpness of public interest in this *curious* announcement is easily understandable. For more than two generations, smallpox inoculation with all its uncertainties and tragic dangers, as well as its cost in time and money, was at least familiar, and though it was still avoided by many physicians and their patients, it had become part of the medical picture and was no longer subject to general interest or discussion. This new vaccination was not only another innovation; it was also ugly and ridiculous. There had been a long tradition — not generally believed, but not forgotten — that all diseases of the infectious sort had come originally from animals, and here was a supposed prevention of infection directly offered from an animal. No, they would have none of it. The response was nearer to indifference than to the anger that had marked the 1721 outbreak.

A few days later, Dr. Waterhouse took the Jenner *Inquiry* and also the Pearson and Woodville reports with him to a meeting of the American Academy of Arts and Sciences of which John Adams, President of the United States, was at that time the president. These gentlemen of the academy were deeply interested. Meanwhile Dr. Waterhouse had written to Dr. Jenner requesting samples of the new vaccine and assuring him of his enthusiastic interest. The six-week back and forth journey being accomplished, the vaccine arrived in good condition. It had been sent in a glass bottle and also on an infected thread.

Dr. Waterhouse immediately did what Zabdiel Boylston and Edward Jenner had done. He inoculated his son, Daniel Oliver Waterhouse, five years old, and on succeeding days: Benjamin, aged three, Mary, aged one, Elizabeth, seven, a twelve-year-old servant boy, and two adults of his household. Everything proceeded according to prediction. The slight illness came on the sixth day; on the seventh and eighth there was a redness in the area where the thread had been inserted; the bluish pustule appeared, corresponding precisely to the illustration Jenner had furnished. The children's illness had been so mild they had scarcely been diverted from their play.

When recovery was complete, Dr. Waterhouse asked Dr. Aspinwall, head of the smallpox hospital in Brookline, to inoculate his patients with smallpox virus to complete the test. He consented, requiring them to be brought to the hospital. This was done and the inoculation proceeded, beginning with the twelve-year-old boy. His arm became infected at the proper time and was very sore. The soreness increased but after two days was completely gone, and there was no trace of smallpox infection anywhere on his body. The same effect was apparent in the other children, who were also inoculated with virus taken from a patient in the hospital. The exclamation of Dr. Waterhouse, who witnessed this effect as Edward Jenner had predicted it, is worth quoting. He said, "One fact, in such cases, is worth a thousand arguments."[1]

As word of this experiment went forth, requests came in for other vaccinations, which Dr. Waterhouse willingly performed. He also wrote many letters to physicians beyond the Boston area, carefully giving the cautions as to the taking of the virus at the proper time, the changes which occurred rendering it ineffective, and to the need for great care on the physician's part — all of which the Jenner

Inquiry makes very plain. Of course, as would surprise no one, these cautions were often disregarded with sad sequels.

Several requests from the south for a supply of the vaccine suggested the wise precaution of putting it in the charge of a responsible physician, and knowing no such person, Dr. Waterhouse wrote first to President Jefferson, who had succeeded Adams as President of the United States. Jefferson's reply was immediate with a name supplied. Dr. Waterhouse at once sent Jefferson a supply of vaccine for his own personal household. It arrived in poor condition as did two subsequent parcels. Summer heat was at its height during these weeks, and Jefferson then suggested that the next supply be sent with the vial of vaccine inserted in a larger container filled with water and that the parcel be sent to Monticello, where the temperature was slightly cooler than Washington, D.C. This was done, the vaccine arrived in good condition, and the President inoculated not only his own family, but also some two hundred of the workers on his plantation. The illustration of the pustule on a dark skin, which Dr. Jenner had thoughtfully supplied, helped to make the vaccination a clearer test.

On November 13, 1799, Dr. Waterhouse wrote a second article in the *Columbian Centinel* which excited a stronger interest in the lay reader as to the possibilities of the new vaccine. "We live in the scrutinizing age of experiment," Waterhouse wrote, "and we cannot doubt that our English brethren will produce a longer chain of facts before we unite in adopting the cowpox vaccine instead of the smallpox virus for our protection." The careless mistakes that were made as soon as it became generally known that protection could be passed from one to another from the single pustule on one's arm caused great alarm among the knowing and hurt the cause of the new discovery severely. Even children vaccinated each other, and a veritable traffic in vaccine led to tragic consequences. An English sailor just off the ship, pretending to be suffering from a cowpox inoculation, was really a smallpox victim. He sold the virus from his own pustules and very soon had caused a minor smallpox outbreak. In

Marblehead the same disaster reached tragic proportions. Many were ill and there were several deaths. In vain Dr. Waterhouse issued one caution after another.

The same situation had of course followed Jenner's first announcement in England. Told of the American parallel, he was deeply distressed, but he knew that only time could prevent such mistakes. Once more he wrote that he wished he had a speaking trumpet that could carry voices across the ocean to announce, "Take the virus before the efflorescence appears." Failure to do so meant there would be no protective action as to smallpox infection. Dr. Boylston had found the same condition to be true for the smallpox virus but had for a long time spoken in vain. By person to person vaccination too long continued, a similar situation arose. Mixing of the lancets was another danger when vaccination was in the hands of the laity. New England experienced all these hazards, over and over.

In 1800 Dr. Waterhouse published *A Prospect of Exterminating Smallpox: being the History of the* Variolae Vaccinae, *or kine-pox, commonly called the cow-pox, Part I.* Part II was issued soon after. These two pamphlets repeat the complete American story since the first announcement by Dr. Waterhouse in the *Columbian Centinel* of July 12, 1799. It still remained to secure some official recognition as to the advantages of this method of protection over the former inoculation with smallpox virus and to make it available to all persons instead of the small fraction able to pay for the elaborate program of preparation demanded by the few in whose hands the practice lay. It had been ten years since an alarm that had led to something like a general inoculation in Boston, and by current estimates there were at least fifteen thousand residents unprotected in case another outbreak should come. The situation looked ominous. "We perceive our houses on fire, and with buckets in our hands, we stand idly gazing into the flames." There had been a time when Edward Jenner, in near desperation, had spoken likewise.

Dr. Waterhouse, feeling a deep sense of duty in this situation and having been rebuffed more than once, decided to try again. This time he appealed to the Board of Health in what he called a *Memorial* dated May 2, 1802.[2] He addressed them as a legally constituted body — twelve men chosen to represent the residents of the town, one from each ward — and charged with keeping watch over the introduction of infection from abroad. Three of them sat daily, superintending and enforcing quarantine and whatever else protected the health of the town. They received no fee for this service. Waterhouse represented himself not as a private inoculator, but as a public teacher in the Commonwealth. In the preceding year he had been appealed to by the Board of Health in connection with quarantine limits in just this capacity, and he used the memory of that service in this *Memorial*. What he was now asking was not patronage for the new vaccine, but rather the conducting of a public experiment that would create confidence and inspire satisfaction. He mentioned a few specifications, but only a few. What he wanted was an affirmative decision in principle.

He got it promptly. Yes, the board would conduct a public experiment that would be decisive. They first built a small building to serve as a hospital on Noddle's Island, one mile from the end of Boston's Long Wharf. They chose seven doctors to serve as inoculators and to make the final examination of the patients. Nineteen boys who had not had the smallpox and had not been inoculated with smallpox virus for protection were chosen as the patients. On August 19 these boys were all inoculated with cowpox virus at the Board of Health office in Boston, the health board being present, as they were at important points through the entire test.

On December 9 twelve of these nineteen boys were inoculated with smallpox virus, supplied by Dr. Aspinwall of the smallpox hospital in Brookline. At the same time two other boys who had not received inoculation either with smallpox or cowpox were also inoculated together with one boy who had been inoculated with cowpox two years before.

At the usual time, the eruptive fever came with pustules. When these pustules were at their highest state of infection, all thirteen children were inoculated a second time, along with the seven boys who had been absent from the first inoculation. All of the children were housed indiscriminately in the same room and indulged in their usual modes of living. No medicines were given at any time. The pustules dried up and disappeared, leaving no sign of smallpox on any of their bodies. The six physicians each examined every child and then signed the paper indicating their satisfaction. The seventh physician, who had not acted throughout the experiment, did not sign. His failure to do so did not mean dissatisfaction, but only that he had had no part in the trial.

The Board of Health announced themselves convinced that cow-pox vaccination was a complete security against smallpox infection and that this experiment was decisive. It had been three years and eight months since Dr. Waterhouse's first article had appeared in the *Columbian Centinel,* and eighty-one years and five months since Dr. Zabdiel Bolyston had inoculated his son Thomas in the great plague year, 1721. Much remained to be done. Many of Boston's population had still to be convinced of the safety of vaccination and of its efficacy in preventing infection. Official legislation making vaccination a federal requirement would meet many snags, but Boston's Board of Health, under the planning of Dr. Waterhouse, had taken an important step toward that final action.

In Benjamin Waterhouse's own words, "This decisive experiment, which has fixed forever the practice of the new experiment in Massachusetts was instituted three years and eight months after my first publication of the existence of such an episodic distemper as the cow-pox and about two years after I made the first experiment with it in America."[3]

Epilogue

NOTABLE ACHIEVEMENTS come in their own way. They are unpredictable, often illogical, and sometimes performed by unlikely agents. Every profession has such chapters. Medical history is full of them. In the present story, Zabdiel Boylston might seem an unlikely man to achieve what is recorded for him. Born and bred a villager, a physician with no academic letters after his name, a man of limited experience in a provincial society, he wrote a distinguished chapter in America's first century of medical history. By his courage, or as his detractors said, by his foolhardy boldness, he dared to try a method of which he had only heard and never witnessed. By his success, which probably surprised him as it surprises us more than two centuries later, he saved many lives and, better still, opened the door for a later man to discover a better method, of which Boylston would never know, and which has not only saved millions more lives, but also has almost exterminated the disease itself. From first to last, Zabdiel Boylston's story is a typical American success story. In fact, his life helped to create the tradition.

Cotton Mather, his Boston neighbor, who started him on his experimental way, was almost his precise opposite in most fundamental ways. He was an intellectual, a man of the printed page who carried a towering freight of knowledge in his head; he had a mind that enabled him also to look beyond the limitations of his time and training, and with an imaginative understanding of quite new ways of thought, to deserve a place at the very beginnings of American scientific observation and interpretation. He stood side by side with Zabdiel Boylston through a day of bitter warfare, as the two men accomplished together what neither of them could have done alone. Theirs was a rare human partnership.

Edward Jenner had the good fortune (for a scientist) to be born nearly a century later, when the light shining on the mystery of man's physical being was beginning to be considerably stronger. He held to a vague and strangely hopeful vision from far earlier times, with a patience and persistence that allowed nothing to defeat him, and in the end he found truth in the laboratory and under the microscope for a folk tradition that hitherto had seemed to merit no serious treatment from the medical profession. In the far-reaching sequel, he won and abundantly deserved the world's acclaim and gratitude. He too opened doors to later men, who are still walking to triumphs he could never have foreseen.

On every working morning of our twentieth century of medical marvels, not hundreds, but thousands of men and women go forth to their laboratories, put on their white coats, feed the research animals, keep the records, and continue the day's disciplined search toward victory over another scourge of many generations.

Notes

Notes

I. AN UNPROFESSIONAL MEDICAL BACKGROUND

1. Massachusetts colonial law, 1649, *Ancient Charters and Laws of Massachusetts Bay*, pp. 76–77. Also in *Laws of Massachusetts* (1672), p. 28.
2. John Evans, Minister, *The Universall Medicine, or the Vertues of the Antimonial Cup* (London: 1634), reprinted in *Proceedings of the Massachusetts Historical Society*, Vol. 60 (1927), pp. 156ff.
3. *Proceedings of the Massachusetts Historical Society*, Vol. 5 (1860–1862), pp. 379–84. For Dr. Oliver Wendell Holmes's comment, see pp. 385–99.
4. Sir Kenelm's Powder, see *Proceedings of the Massachusetts Historical Society*, Vol. 59 (1925), pp. 87–92.
5. Mentioned by Francis Brown, "The Practice of Medicine in New England before 1700," *Bostonian Society Publications*, Vol. 8 (1911), pp. 104–5.

II. A HALF CENTURY OF PASTOR-PHYSICIANS

1. Brief mention only, in Salem *Annals*, 2 vols. (1845), Salem, Mass.; in Wilson Waters, *History of Chelmsford, Massachusetts* (1917), Lowell, Mass., p. 17.
2. *Colonial Society Publications*, Vol. 19, pp. 274, 275.
3. General Court Records, Vol. 2, p. 175, quoted in *Proceedings of the Massachusetts Historical Society*, 2nd ser., Vol. 1, pp. 46–47.
4. See Illustration below.
5. First published in 1662 and reissued many times since. A modern-

ized reprint of the first edition was published by W. H. Burr and J. W. Dean in 1867. A more recent reprint was edited by K. B. Murdock in 1929.

6. *The Poetical Works of Edward Taylor* was edited with an Introduction and Notes by Thomas H. Johnson, who discovered the manuscript in 1939. "Meditation 62" is on page 169.

7. *Will and Doom* is printed in the *Connecticut Historical Society Collections,* Vol. 92 (1714) by W. R. Steiner.

8. Extant materials concerning Jared Eliot have been collected by Herbert Thoms under the title *Jared Eliot, Minister, Doctor, Scientist, and His Connecticut* (1967).

III. FIVE MAJOR OUTBREAKS IN ONE LIFETIME SPAN

1. For this early stage estimates differ. Dr. Jurin's were compiled not only from Bills of Mortality, but in direct correspondence with physicians of the area.

2. *The Historical Magazine* (Boston: August 1857), pp. 228–31. See also Green, *Facsimile Reproductions* (Boston: 1901).

3. Diary, *Collections of the Massachusetts Historical Society,* 7th ser., Vol. 8, p. 451.

4. Sidney Perley, *The History of Salem* (Salem: 1924), pp. 128–29. Quoted, with slightly different spelling, in *Proceedings of the Massachusetts Historical Society,* 2nd ser., Vol. 1 (1884), p. 47.

5. *Records of Newbury,* September 28, 1638.

IV. FIRST HOPE FROM FAR PLACES

1. Diary, *Collections of the Massachusetts Historical Society,* Vol. 7, December 15, 1706/1707, p. 579.

2. *Philosophical Transactions of the Royal Society,* Vol. 29 (London: 1717), pp. 71–82.

3. George Lyman Kittredge, "Lost Works of Cotton Mather," *Proceedings of the Massachusetts Historical Society,* Vol. 45 (1912), p. 422.

4. *Philosophical Transactions,* Vol. 29, pp. 393–99, in Latin.

5. Unpublished, recorded, grouped, annotated by George Lyman Kittredge, under the title "Cotton Mather's Scientific Contributions to the Royal Society," *American Antiquarian Society Proceedings,* Vol. 26 (1916), pp. 18–57.

6. *The Angel of Bethesda* (Worcester: 1972), p. 94. "It begins to be vehemently suspected that the S . . . . P . . may be more of an Animalculated Business than we have been generally aware of. The Millions of ——— which the Microscopes discover have Confirmed this Suspicion." This suggestion of the germ theory is believed to be the earliest in America. Mather's *Angel of Bethesda* remained in manuscript until 1972.

7. Rhazes, Arabian physician. His title, *A Treatise on the Smallpox or Measles,* translated by Richard Mead, *The Medical Works of Richard Mead* (Edinburgh: 1775).

8. G. L. Kittredge, "Lost Works of C. M." *Proceedings of the Massachusetts Historical Society,* Vol. 95, p. 422.

9. Diary, *Collections of the Massachusetts Historical Society,* Vol. 7, p. 621. After May 26, 1721, diary entries are in Vol. 8.

V. ONE PRACTITIONER FOR EACH THOUSAND RESIDENTS

1. "Letters from Dr. William Douglass to Cadwallader Colden of New York," *Collections of the Massachusetts Historical Society,* 4th ser., Vol. 2 (1854), pp. 164–89.

2. Abner Morse, *A Genealogical Record,* Chapter 1 gives a brief statement of fact as to Cutler. George M. Bodge records his service in King Philip's War in *Soldiers in King Philip's War* (Boston: 1891).

3. There is no biography of Zabdiel Boylston and extant records out of which a biography might be written are apparently lacking. We know him chiefly from local references during the smallpox siege of 1721.

4. A brief sketch of Douglass written by Charles D. Bullock entitled "Life and Writings of William Douglass" appears in *Economic Studies,* Vol. 112, pp. 265–90.

VI. BOSTON'S GREAT PLAGUE YEAR, 1721

1. Diary, *Collections of the Massachusetts Historical Society,* May 26, 1721, pp. 620–21.
2. *Ibid.,* p. 628. The letter is dated June 6, 1721.
3. *Ibid.,* Diary entry of March 13, 1717, Vol. 7, p. 523.
4. Reprinted in the *Massachusetts Magazine,* Vol. 1 (1789), with two other letters, pp. 776–79.
5. Diary, *Collections of the Massachusetts Historical Society,* July and August 1721. Day after day another aspect of this "clamour," pp. 631, 632.
6. Zabdiel Boylston reprinted the three Instances at the conclusion of his *Historical Account* (London: 1726), Appendix, pp. 51–53.
7. Under "A Few Quaeries humbly Offered," *An Account of Inoculating or Transplanting the Small Pox* (1721), pp. 10–11.
8. Zabdiel Boylston's statement of these totals appears at the end of his *Historical Account* with tables, pp. 34–35.

VII. ENGLAND'S PROMOTER OF INOCULATION WAS A TITLED LADY

1. Charles Maitland's *Account of Inoculating the Small-Pox* (London: 1722).
2. Robert Halsband, *The Life of Mary Wortley Montagu* (Oxford: 1966), p. 51. Also in *Complete Letters,* Vol. 1, pp. 338–39.
3. To Edward Wortley, *Complete Works of Lady Mary Wortley Montagu,* Vol. 1, pp. 392, 393. See also Halsband, *Life,* p. 81.
4. Edmund Massey's final word to his readers who are not satisfied with his warnings is that they consult Dr. Wagstaffe's *Letter to Dr. Friend.*
5. Halsband, *Life,* p. 111.

VIII. ZABDIEL BOYLSTON IN LONDON

1. It was recommended for aches, bruises, sprains.
2. For various background details see Raymond P. Stearns, "Colonial Fellows of the Royal Society," *William and Mary Quarterly,* 3rd ser. (April 1946).

3. From the *Obligation* signed by each newly elected member after being admitted.

4. Thomas Robie, whose election immediately preceded Boylston's, had also a few Boston patients during 1721 for inoculation.

5. The *Philosophical Transactions* did not print an account of his second gift, a large stone found in the stomach of a horse, but the letter in which Sir Hans Sloane acknowledged the specimen is preserved. It was dated December 28, 1727, and was most apologetic for the long delay.

6. Quoted from the *New England Historical and Genealogical Society's Register,* Vol. 35, p. 129, to which Ward Nicholas Boylston probably sent it himself. It deserves another printing.

IX. ZABDIEL BOYLSTON'S *An Historical Account,* 1726

1. Boylston, *An Historical Account,* 1726, p. 2.
2. *Ibid.,* pp. 5–6.
3. *Ibid.,* pp. 25–27. He had found the Indian girl sitting up in bed, entirely unclothed. She had caught cold, the Pock had sunk in; many Means were used to bring the Pock out again, but to no purpose, for she died before Morning.
4. *Ibid.,* p. 21.
5. *Ibid.,* pp. 22–23.
6. *Ibid.,* pp. 32–33.

X. WAR OF WORDS

1. Diary entry of June 22, 1721. This was four days before Boylston's first operation.
2. Published in London, 1721.
3. This tract was published also in London and Dublin.
4. Possibly as late as September 1721. He had deliberately waited to gain perspective before speaking.
5. Ministers "going out of their way" to engage in this debate had been one of the most persistent criticisms of them through all these months.

6. At this early date Colman was one of the very few to speak this affirmatively on the positive side of the argument.

7. This tract also was published in England.

8. Published February 5, 1722.

9. *Vindication,* p. 2.

10. Diary, *Collections of the Massachusetts Historical Society,* Vol. 8, January 19, January 25–26, 1721/1722, pp. 672, 674.

11. Douglass, William, *A Dissertation Concerning Inoculation of the Smallpox* (London: 1730) p. 63.

XI. TWO GENERATIONS OF DOUBTFUL PRACTICE

1. The full story of Salem's unhappy affair is told by Gerard H. Clarfield in an article, "Salem's Great Inoculation Controversy, 1773–1774," *Essex Institute Historical Collections,* Vol. 106 (Salem, Mass.: October 1970), pp. 277–96.

2. The Marblehead story, recalled by a modern scholar, George A. Billias, is also published in the *E. I. H. Collections,* under the title "Pox and Politics in Marblehead, 1773–1774," Vol. 92 (1956), pp. 43–58.

XII. EDWARD JENNER'S *Inquiry,* 1798

1. At the end of *An Inquiry into Cause and Effects of the* Variolae Vaccinae.

2. The best way to know Edward Jenner as a man in his time is through his life story, written by John Baron, who knew him personally and kept always before him, in spite of long tangential episodes, the importance of his great discovery. The book was published in two volumes in London in 1838. Another later book, brief but carefully written, is Dorothy Fisk's *Dr. Jenner of Berkeley* (London: 1957). Naturally, there is a veritable library of discussion concerning his discovery for the specialist of which this present sketch can take no account.

XIII. BENJAMIN WATERHOUSE'S CAMPAIGN IN BOSTON

1. Benjamin Waterhouse, *A Prospect of Exterminating the Smallpox: being the History of the* Variolae Vaccinae, *or kine-pox, commonly called the cow pox* (Cambridge, Mass.: 1800), p. 25. Part II, printed immediately following and also separately under the title *Progress of the New Inoculation in America* (Cambridge: 1802).

2. Waterhouse, *A Prospect of Exterminating the Smallpox,* Part I, pp. 51–53.

3. *Ibid.,* pp. 64–65, 73.

Bibliography

Bibliography

Baron, John. *The Life of Edward Jenner,* 2 vols. London, 1838.

Bartlett, Josiah. *A Dissertation on the Progress of Medical Science in Massachusetts.* Boston, 1810.

Beall, Otho T., and Shyrock, Richard H. "Cotton Mather, First Significant Figure in American Medicine." *Proceedings of the American Antiquarian Society,* Vol. 63 (1953), pp. 37–274.

Bell, Whitfield. "Medical Practice in Colonial America." In *Symposium on Colonial Medicine.* Wiilliamsburg, Virginia, 1957.

Billias, George A. "Pox and Politics in Marblehead 1773–1774." *Essex Institute Historical Collections,* Vol. 92 (1956), pp. 43–58.

Blake, John B. "The Inoculation Controversy in Boston, 1721–1722." *New England Quarterly,* Vol. 25 (1952), pp. 484–506.

———. *Public Health in the Town of Boston, 1630–1832.* Cambridge, Mass.: Harvard University Press, 1959.

Blanton, Wyndham B. *Medicine in Virginia in the Eighteenth Century.* Richmond, 1931.

Bond, Henry. *Genealogies of the Families and Descendants of the Early Settlers of Watertown.* Boston, 1860. (See Boylston.)

Boorstin, Daniel Joseph. *The Americans, the Colonial Experience.* New York, 1954, 1958, 1965.

———. *The National Experience.* New York, 1965.

Boston *Courant.* August 1721–March 1722.

Boston *Gazette.* May 1721–May 1722.

Boston News Letter. May 1721–May 1722.

Boylston, Zabdiel. "Ambergris Found in Whales." *Philosophical Transactions of the Royal Society,* Vol. 33 (1726).

———. *An Historical Account of the Small Pox Inoculated in New England.* London, 1726. Reprinted, Boston, 1730.

Brasch, Frederick. "The Royal Society of London and Its Influence upon Scientific Thought in the American Colonies." *Scientific Monthly,* Vol. 33 (1931), pp. 337–55.

Brooks, E. St. John. *Sir Hans Sloane, the Great Collector and His Circle.* London, 1954.

Brown, Francis H. M. D. "The Practice of Medicine in New England Before 1700." *Bostonian Society Publications,* Vol. 8 (1911), pp. 104–5.

Bullock, Charles D. "Life and Writings of William Douglass." *Economic Studies,* Vol. 112, pp. 265–90.

Burrage, W. L. *A History of the Massachusetts Medical Society, with Brief Biographies,* 1781, 1922, 1953.

Clarfield, Gerard H. "Salem's Great Inoculation Controversy, 1773–1774." *Essex Institute Historical Collections,* Vol. 103 (1910).

Clark, George M. "Jacobean England, 1692–1725." In *Symposium on Colonial Medicine.* Williamsburg, Virginia, 1957.

Colman, Benjamin. "Some Observations on the New Method of Receiving the Smallpox by Engrafting or Inoculation, in New England." Boston, 1721.

Culpepper, Nicholas. *A Physical Directory.* London, 1649.

Cooper, William. *A Letter to a Friend in the Country.* Boston, 1721.

Curiosa Americana. (See Kittredge.)

Douglass, William. *A Dissertation Concerning Inoculation of the Smallpox.* London, 1730.

———. *A Practical Essay Concerning the Smallpox.* Boston, 1730.

Duffy, John. *Epidemics in Colonial America.* Baton Rouge, 1953.

Figuier, Louis. *Vies des Servants du Moyen Age.* Paris, 1867. (See Rhazes, pp. 43–54.)

Fisk, Dorothy. *Dr. Jenner of Berkeley.* London, 1957.

Fitz, Reginald H. "Zabdiel Boylston, Inoculator, and the Epidemic of Smallpox in Boston in 1721." *Bulletin of the Johns Hopkins Hospital,* Vol. 22 (1911), no. 247, pp. 315–27.

Greenwood, Isaac. *A Friendly Debate or a Dialogue between Academicus and Sawny and Mundungus.* Boston, 1721–1722.

Guerra, Francis. *American Medical Bibliography.* New York, 1962.

Halsband, Robert. *The Life of Mary Wortley Montague.* Oxford, 1966. Rev. 1967.

Hamilton, Bernice. "The Medical Professions in the 18th Century." *Economic Historical Review* (1961), pp. 141–69.

Jenner, Edward. *An Inquiry into the Causes and Effects of* Variolae Vaccinae *or Cow-Pox.* London, 1798.

———. "Origin of the *Vaccinae* Inoculation." *Philosophical Transactions of the Royal Society,* Vol. 32, p. 214.

Kelly, Howard A., and Burrage, Walter L. *Dictionary of American Medical Biographies.* New York, 1928.

Kiligrew, F. G. "The Rise of Scientific Activity in Colonial New England." *Yale Journal of Biology and Medicine* (1949), pp. 123–38.

King, Lester S. *The Medical World of the Eighteenth Century.* Chicago, 1956.

Kittredge, George Lyman. "Lost Works of Cotton Mather." *Proceedings of the Massachusetts Historical Society,* Vol. 45 (1912), pp. 418–79.

————. "Cotton Mather's Contributions to the Royal Society." *American Antiquarian Society Proceedings,* Vol. 26, 1916, pp. 18–57.

Introduction to Increase Mather's *Several Reasons.* Cotton Mather's *Sentiments on the Smallpox Inoculated.*

Klebs, Arnold C. "Historic Evolution of Variolation." *Bulletin of the Johns Hopkins Hospital,* Vol. 24 (1913), no. 265, pp. 69–83.

Lettsom, Benjamin. *Observations on Cow-Pock.* London, 1801.

Long, Henry. "The Physicians of Topsfield." *Essex Institute Historical Collections.*

Massey, Edmund. *The Dangerous and Sinful Practice of Inoculation,* 2nd ed. London, 1730.

Mather, Cotton. Diary, 1631–1708, 1709–1724. *Collections of the Massachusetts Historical Society,* Vol. 7, 8, 7th ser.

————. *The Angel of Bethesda.* An essay on the common maladies of mankind. Barre, Mass., 1972.

Middlekopf, Robert. *The Mathers, Three Generations of Puritan Intellectuals.* New York, 1971.

Montagu, Lady Mary Wortley. *The Complete Works of Lady Mary Wortley Montagu,* 3 vols. London, 1965–1967.

Moore, Francis D., M.D. "Therapeutic Innovation: Ethical Boundaries to the Initial Clinical Trials of New Drugs and Surgical Procedures." *Daedalus, Journal of the American Academy of Arts and Sciences,* Vol. 98, Spring 1969, pp. 502–22.

Morison, Samuel Eliot. *The Intellectual Life of Colonial New England.* New York, 1956.

Mumford, James Gregory. *A Narrative of Medicine in America.* Philadelphia and London, 1903.

Pettigrew, Thomas Joseph. *The Superstitions Connected with the History and Practice of Medicine and Surgery.* Philadelphia, 1844.

Prince, Thomas. *Annals of New England.* Boston, 1736.

Pylarinus, Jacobus. *"Nova & Tuta Variolas Excitandi per Transplantationem Methodus Nuper Inventa & in Usum Tracta."* *Philosophical Transactions of the Royal Society,* Vol. 29 (1714), no. 347, pp. 393–99.

Osler, Sir William. *The Evolution of Modern Medicine.* New Haven, 1921.

Sewall, Samuel. Diary. *Collections of the Massachusetts Historical Society,* 3 vols., 5th ser., 1878, 1879, 1882.

Shyrock, R. H. *Medicine and Society in America.* New York, 1960.

————. "Eighteenth Century Medicine in America." *American Antiquarian Society Collections,* Vol. 109.

————. *Medicine in America.* Baltimore, 1966.

Stearns, Raymond P. "Colonial Fellows of the Royal Society of London." *William and Mary Quarterly,* 3rd ser., 1946, pp. 208–68.

Thacher, James. *American Medical Biography,* 2 vols. Boston, 1828.

Thacher, Thomas. *A Brief Rule to Guide the Common People of New England.* Boston, 1677.

Timonius, Emanuel. "An Account, or History, of the Procuring the Small Pox by Incision, or Inoculation." *Philosophical Transactions of the Royal Society,* Vol. 29 (1714), no. 339, pp. 73–82.

Toner, Joseph M. *Contributions to the Annals of Medical Progress and Medical Education in the United States Before and During the War of Independence.* Washington, 1874.

Viets, Henry R. *A Brief History of Medicine in Massachusetts.* Boston, 1930.

Waterhouse, Benjamin. *A Prospect of Exterminating the Smallpox.* Cambridge, Mass., 1800.

———. *Progress of the New Inoculation in America.* Cambridge, Mass., 1802.

Woodville, William. *The History of the Inoculation of the Small-pox in Great Britain,* 1802.

Index

Index